Mathematical Tables: Containing The Common, Hyperbolic, And Logistic Logarithms...

Charles Hutton

MATHEMATICAL TABLES.

Printed by S. Hamilton, Weybridge.

MATHEMATICAL TABLES;

CONTAINING THE

COMMON, HYPERBOLIC, AND LOGISTIC

LOGARITHMS,

ALSO

SINES, TANGENTS, SECANTS, & VERSED SINES

BOTH NATURAL AND LOGARITHMIC.

TOGETHER WITH

SEVERAL OTHER TABLES

USEFUL IN

MATHEMATICAL CALCULATIONS.

To which is prefixed,

A LARGE AND ORIGINAL HISTORY OF THE DISCOVERIES AND WRITINGS
RELATING TO THOSE SUBJECTS;

WITH THE

COMPLETE DESCRIPTION AND USE OF THE TABLES.

◆——◆

THE FIFTH EDITION.

◆——◆

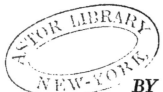

BY CHARLES HUTTON,

LL.D. F.R.S. &c.

AND LATE PROFESSOR OF MATHEMATICS IN THE ROYAL MILITARY ACADEMY,
WOOLWICH.

LONDON:

PRINTED FOR F. C. AND J. RIVINGTON; WILKIE AND ROBINSON;
J. WALKER; LACKINGTON, ALLEN, AND CO.; VERNOR, HOOD, AND
SHARPE; C. LAW; LONGMAN, HURST, REES, ORME, AND BROWN;
BLACK, PARRY, AND KINGSBURY; J. RICHARDSON; L. B. SEELEY;
J. MURRAY; R. BALDWIN; SHERWOOD, NEELY, AND JONES; GALE
AND CURTIS; J. JOHNSON AND CO.; AND G. ROBINSON.
1811.

PREFACE.

━━━

THE very ample introduction, prefixed to the following collection of Mathematical Tables, supersedes the necessity of using many words here by way of preface, and leaves little more to be mentioned than the necessity and occasion of this work, with some account of the contents and mode of execution.

The undertaking was occasioned by the great incorrectness of all the editions of Sherwin's or Gardiner's tables, and more especially by the bad arrangement in the fifth or last edition. Finding, as well from the report of others, as from my own experience, that those editions (to say nothing of the very improper alteration in the form of the table of sines, tangents, and secants in the last of them) were so very incorrectly printed, the errors being multiplied beyond all tolerable bounds, and no dependence to be placed on them for any thing of real practice, I was led to undertake the painful office of preparing a correct edition of another similar work. And I was lucky enough to meet with a bookseller of sufficient spirit to be at the great expense of printing the book, as well as to allow me what I demanded for my trouble in preparing it; which demand, however, was nothing adequate to the great labour attending it, as I was well aware that the profits of the book would not enable him fully to reward my pains.

I have in the first place, therefore, used all the means in my power to render the work correct. I began by collating the third or best edition of Sherwin's tables, with some others of the most perfect works of the same kind, as Briggs's, Vlacq's, Gardiner's quarto book, &c; by which means I detected many errors in each of them, which had not before been discovered; and of these, between twenty and thirty were in the two editions of Gardiner's quarto work, printed at London in 1742, and at Avignon in 1770; the errata of which two books are here printed at the end of the tables in this work. But, besides detecting many unknown errors in the said third edition of Sherwin, which was no more than was expected, I discovered, with no small surprise, that the last figures in the table of logarithms were not uniformly true to the nearest unit, except in a very few pages at the beginning and end of the table; though Mr. Gardiner, the editor of that edition, had made the table correct in that respect in his own quarto work before mentioned, which was also printed in the same year 1742, with the said third edition of Sherwin! The errors from this cause, in that third edition, amounted to several thousands; and they have continued to run through all the editions of Sherwin ever since that time! But they are here corrected. Nor has less attention been employed in correcting the press, than in previously correcting the copy; every proof having been several times read over, and compared with the best of the books hitherto printed, by several persons attending to the reading of every proof-sheet.

But in giving this edition to the world, I was not satisfied with barely making it correct. I was aware that the materials themselves might be much improved; and I have accordingly enlarged, or otherwise greatly amended them, in various respects. Among the improvements of the old materials may be reckoned the following :—namely, in the large table of logarithms, the proportional parts, near the beginning, are more conveniently arranged, being now all placed in the same opening of the book where their corresponding differences occur; the logarithms to sixty-one figures are brought to their proper place in the book, and more conveniently disposed all in one page; the large table of sines, tangents, and secants, is more commodiously arranged, and rendered more distinct and convenient for use; the natural sines, tangents, secants, and versed sines, being all separated from the others, and placed all together on the left-hand pages, and the logarithmic ones facing them on the right-hand pages; the common differences, in both, set between the two columns to which each of them answers; and the versed sines here introduced into their proper place in the same pages with the sines, tangents, and secants. Besides these, there are some other alterations in the new tables here given, and the reader will find a number of very important improvements in the description and use of the whole; especially in the arithmetic of logarithms, and in the resolution of plane and spherical triangles, according to the present improved methods of calculation used by the Astronomer Royal, and other persons the most experienced in these matters.

The improvements in the tables, by the introduction of new matter, are both great and numerous. The tables numbered 2, 3, and 4, are here added, being an entire new set, with their differences, for finding numbers and logarithms to twenty places. The columns of common differences, in the pages of natural sines, &c, are now first introduced: As are also the tables of hyperbolic and logistic logarithms; the logarithmic sines and tangents for every second, in the first two degrees of the quadrant; together with a table of the length of arcs, a table to change common and hyperbolic logarithms from the one to the other, &c.—the uses and exemplifications of the whole being very amply detailed.

But the greatest alteration of all is the very extensive and new introduction here given, instead of the former inadequate and heterogeneous one, consisting of about 180 pages of new matter, on a methodical plan, containing the historical account and description of all trigonometrical writings, and the tables relating to that subject, both natural and logarithmic; besides the complete use of the tables in this work. Inventions are here ascribed to the proper authors, and their methods and improvements described and compared. This historical description will evidently appear to be the result of immense labour and reading. And, indeed, I have painfully gone over all the books which are here so minutely described; and that description with a detail in some degree adequate to their great merits; especially the works of Napier, Briggs, Kepler, &c; which was the more necessary, as the writings and methods of those great masters had not been any where properly described and discriminated, though they are in themselves highly curious and important.

These readings and commentaries have been carried on to an extent far beyond what was at first intended. But the tables having been in the press for the space of seven or eight years, I had thereby an opportunity of collecting and examining a still greater number of books; so that I was gradually led on, and my views and plans rendered still more extensive and complete. This delay, therefore, though in many respects it proved very inconvenient and disagreeable, has at length been the occasion of rendering these commentaries more perfect and satisfactory.

Besides what immediately relates to trigonometrical subjects, the reader will here find many other curious and uncommon articles, relating to their several authors and their discoveries, which have occurred in the course of my reading, and which appeared of too much consequence to be passed over unnoticed, in the analysis of their several compositions. Among these, is the discovery of the first author of the binomial theorem, and the differential method, which are due to Mr. Henry Briggs, whose writings are replete with ingenious and original matter, and are well deserving to be more generally known and studied than they have been for some time past.

This long course of examination and description, however, having been carried on for so many years, at different intervals, and interrupted by various avocations, and by business of different kinds, it will be no wonder if this circumstance may have occasioned some inequalities in the style and composition of this history; and for which, therefore, should any such appear, it is hoped the occasion will plead an apology.

WOOLWICH,
Feb. 1785.

*** IN the large table of common logarithms, when the first of the last four figures in any logarithm changes from a 9 to a 0, in any line, in which case the first three or constant figures are prefixed to the next following line, instead of these three, it often happens that young beginners by mistake take out the three constant figures next above the said line. To guard against this error, the figures in this edition are so contrived, that where the said change happens, a bar is placed over the cipher, thus $\bar{0}$, in order to catch the eye, and remind the learner that the change there takes place.——In this edition, too, the black rules formerly drawn across the pages, at the intervals of every five, or six, or ten lines, have been taken out, leaving thin white spaces across the pages instead of them. These improvements, besides that of new and better formed figures here now introduced, and other attentions, contribute to render this edition of the tables more convenient and correct than either of the former ones.

C. H.
Dec. 1800.

———◆———

IN this *fifth edition*, several of the tables have been much enlarged and improved, and some new ones introduced. Thus, the first large table of logarithms, which heretofore extended only to 100000 numbers, is now enlarged by one whole sheet more, being continued to 108000 numbers. Also the tables on pages 196, 199, 202, 216, are all extended to more numbers than formerly. A new and extensive table of Hyperbolic Logarithms is introduced after the old one ending page 211. The lists of errors, discovered in the best books of logarithms, that have been printed in this country and elsewhere, are more enlarged and corrected. By all which improvements, this collection of tables is rendered much more useful and valuable, than any of the former editions.

London,
May 1811.

———————————————————

Errata, *in the Introduction.*

Page 121, line 21, for Lansihangel, read Lanfihangel.
128, — 17, for log. $\frac{1}{2}$, read log. $\frac{1}{4}$.
149, — 4 from the bot. for x1, read x—1.
157, — 5 from the bot. for $s.\frac{1}{2}.\overline{A+B}$, read $s.\frac{1}{4}.\overline{A+B}$.

In the Tables.

264, Nat. Tan. 8° 1′ should be 1408375.
265, Log. Vers. 8 22 ——— 8·0270578.
271, L. Covers. 11 52 ——— 9·9000202.
337, Log. Tan. 44 60 ——— 10·0000000.

Additional Errata in the French Tables of 1801.

In the logs. to 61 places, No. 14, col. 5, for 12992, read 12922.

In the Logistic Logarithms.

80′ 60″, for 8696, read 8697.
85 31, — 8481, — 8461.
85 33, — 8469, — 8459.

A short Abstract of the principal Contents, may be as follows:

1. *In the Introduction.*

2. *In the Tables themselves.*

INTRODUCTION.

======

I. OF TRIGONOMETRICAL TABLES.

NECESSITY, the fruitful mother of most useful inventions, gave birth to the various numeral tables which compose the following work. Astronomy has been cultivated from the earliest ages. The progress of that science, requiring numerous arithmetical computations of the sides and angles of triangles, both plane and spherical, gave rise to trigonometry; for those frequent calculations suggested the necessity of performing them by the property of similar triangles; and for the ready application of this property, it was necessary that certain lines described in and about circles, to a determinate radius, should be computed, and disposed. in tables. Navigation, and the continually improving accuracy of astronomy, have also occasioned as perpetual an increase in the accuracy and extent of those tables. And this it is evident must ever be the case, the improvement of trigonometry uniformly following the improvement of those other useful sciences, for the sake of which it is more especially cultivated.

The ancients performed their trigonometry by means of the chords of arcs, which, with the chords of their supplemental arcs, and the constant diameter, formed all species of right-angled triangles. Beginning with the radius, and the arc whose chord is equal to the radius, they divided them both into 60 equal parts, and estimated all other arcs and chords by those parts, namely, all arcs by 60ths of that arc, and all chords by 60ths of its chord or of the radius. At least this method is as old as the writings of Ptolemy, who used the sexagenary arithmetic for this division of chords and arcs, and for astronomical purposes.—And this, by-the-by, may be the reason why the whole circumference is divided into 360, or 6 times 60, equal parts or degrees, the whole circumference being equal to 6 times the first arc, whose chord is equal to the radius: unless perhaps we are rather to seek for the division of the circle in the number of days in the year; for thus, the ancient year consisting of 360 days, the sun or earth in each day described the 360th part of the orbit; and thence might arise the method of dividing every circle into 360 parts; and radius being equal to the chord of 60 of those parts, the sexagesimal division, both of the radius and of the parts, might thence arise. Trigonometry however must have been cultivated long before the time of Ptolemy; and indeed Theon, in his commentary on

B

Ptolemy's Almagest, l. i. ch. 9., mentions a work of the philosopher Hipparchus, written about a century and a half before Christ, consisting of 12 books on the chords of circular arcs: which must have been a treatise on trigonometry. And Menelaus also, in the first century of Christ, wrote 6 books concerning subtenses or chords of arcs. He used the word *nadir* (of an arc), which he defined to be the right line subtending the double of the arc; so that his nadir of an arc was the double of our sine of the same arc, or the chord of the double arc; and therefore whatever he proves of the former, may be applied to the latter, substituting the double sine for the nadir.

The radius has been since decimally divided; but the sexagesimal divisions of the arc have continued in use to this day. Indeed our countrymen, Briggs and Gellibrand, having a general dislike to all sexagesimal divisions, made an attempt at some reformation of this custom, by dividing the degrees of the arcs, in their tables, into centesms or hundredth parts, instead of minutes or 60th parts. The same was also recommended by Vieta, and others; and a decimal division of the whole quadrant* might perhaps soon have followed, had it not been for the tables of Vlacq, which came out a little after, to every 10 seconds, or 6th parts of a minute.—But the complete reformation would be, to express all arcs by their real lengths, namely, in equal parts of the radius decimally divided: according to which method I have nearly completed a table of sines and tangents.

It is not to be doubted that many of the ancients wrote on the subject of trigonometry, as being a necessary part of astronomy; though few of their labours on that branch have come to our knowledge, and still fewer of the writings themselves have been handed down to us. We are in possession of the three books of Menelaus, on spherical trigonometry; but the six books are lost which he wrote upon chords, being probably a treatise on the construction of trigonometrical tables.

The trigonometry of Menelaus was much improved by Ptolemy (Claudius Ptolomæus) the celebrated philosopher and mathematician. He was born at Pelusium, taught astronomy at Alexandria in Egypt, and died in the year of Christ 147, being the 78th year of his age. In the first book of his Almagest, Ptolemy delivers a table of arcs and chords, with the method of construction. This table contains 3 columns; in the first are the arcs to every half degree or 30 minutes; in the 2d are their chords, expressed in degrees, minutes and seconds, of which degrees the radius contains 60; and in the 3d column are the differences of the chords answering to 1 minute of the arcs, or the 30th part of the differences between the chords in the 2d column. In the construction of this table, among others, Ptolemy shows, for the first time that we know of, this property of any quadrilateral inscribed in a circle, namely, that the rectangle under the two diagonals, is equal to the sum of the two rectangles under the opposite sides.

This method of computation, by the chords, continued in use till about the middle centuries after Christ; when it was changed for that of the sines, which were about that time introduced into trigonometry

---

* This has lately been done by the French mathematicians, in their new logarithmic tables.

by the Arabians, who in other respects much improved this science, which they had received from the Greeks, introducing, among other things, the three or four theorems, or axioms, which are used at present as the foundation of our modern trigonometry.

. The other great improvements that have been made in this branch, are due to the Europeans. These improvements they have gradually introduced since they received this science from the Arabians. And though these latter people had long used the Indian or decimal scale of arithmetic, it does not appear that they varied from the Greek or sexagesimal division of the radius, by which the chords and sines were expressed.

This alteration, it is said, was first made by George Purbach, who was so called from his being a native of a place of that name between Austria and Bavaria. He was born in 1423, studied mathematics and astronomy at the university of Vienna, where he was afterwards professor of those sciences, though but for a short time, the learned world quickly suffering a great loss by his immature death, which happened in 1462, at the age of 39 years only. Purbach, besides enriching trigonometry and astronomy with several new tables, theorems, and observations, supposed the radius to be divided into 600,000 equal parts, and computed the sines of the arcs, for every 10 minutes, in such equal parts of the radius, by the decimal notation.

This project of Purbach was completed by his disciple, companion, and successor, John Muller, or Regiomontanus, who was so called from the place of his nativity, the little town of Mons Regius, or Koningsberg, in Franconia, where he was born in the year 1436. Regiomontanus not only extended the sines to every minute, the radius being 600,000, as designed by Purbach, but afterwards, disliking that scheme as evidently imperfect, he computed them likewise to the radius 1,000,000, for every minute of the quadrant. He also introduced the tangents into trigonometry, the canon of which he called *fœcundus*, because of the many and great advantages arising from them. Besides these, he enriched trigonometry with many theorems and precepts. Through the benefit of all these improvements, except for the use of logarithms, the trigonometry of Regiomontanus is but little inferior to that of our own time. His treatise on both plane and spherical trigonometry, is in 5 books; it was written about the year 1464, and printed in folio at Nuremburg, in 1533. And in the fifth book are also various problems concerning rectilinear triangles, some of which are resolved by means of algebra: a proof that this science was not wholly unknown in Europe before the treatise of Lucas de Burgo. Regiomontanus died in 1476, at the age of 40 years only; being then at Rome, whither he had been invited by the Pope, to assist in the reformation of the Calendar, and where it was suspected he was poisoned by the sons of George Trebizonde, in revenge for the death of their father, which was said to have been caused by the grief he felt on account of the criticisms made by Regiomontanus on his translation of Ptolemy's Almagest.

Soon after this, several other mathematicians contributed to the improvement of trigonometry, by extending and enlarging the tables, though few of their works have been printed; and particularly John Werner of Nuremburg, who was born in 1468, and died in 1528, and who it seems wrote five books on triangles.

About the year 1500, Nicholas Copernicus, the celebrated modern restorer of the true solar system, wrote a brief treatise on trigonometry, both plane and spherical, with the description and construction of the canon of chords, or their halves, nearly in the manner of Ptolemy; to which is subjoined a canon of sines, with their differences, for every 10 minutes of the quadrant, to the radius 100,000. This tract is inserted in the first book of his *Revolutiones Orbium Cælestium*, first printed in folio at Nuremburg, 1543. It is remarkable that he does not call these lines *sines*, but *semisses subtensarum*, namely of the double arcs.— Copernicus was born at Thorn in 1473, and died in 1543.

In 1553 was published the *Canon Fœcundus*, or table of tangents, of Erasmus Reinhold, professor of mathematics in the academy of Wurtemburgh. He was born at Salfieldt in Upper Saxony, in the year 1511, and died in 1553.

To Francis Maurolyc, abbot of Messina in Sicily, we owe the introduction of the *Tabula Benefica*, or canon of secants, which came out about the same time, or a little before. But Lansberg erroneously ascribes this to Rheticus. And the tangents and secants are both ascribed to Reinhold, by Briggs, in his *Mathematica ab antiquis minus cognita*, (p. 80. Appendix to Ward's Lives of the Professors of Gresham College.)

Francis Vieta was born in 1540, at Fontenai, or Fontenai-le-Comte, in Lower Poitou, a province of France. He was master of requests at Paris, where he died in 1603, being the 63d year of his age. Among other branches of learning in which he excelled, he was one of the most respectable mathematicians of the 16th century, or indeed of any age. His writings abound with marks of great originality, and the finest genius, as well as intense application. Among them are several pieces relating to trigonometry, which may be found in the collection of his works published at Leyden in 1646, by Francis Schooten, besides another large and separate volume in folio, published in the author's lifetime at Paris in 1579, containing trigonometrical tables, with their construction and use; very elegantly printed, by the king's mathematical printer, with beautiful types and rules: the differences of the sines, tangents, and secants, and some other parts, being printed with red ink, for the better distinction; but inaccurately executed, as he himself testifies in page 323 of his other works above mentioned. The first part of this curious volume is entitled *Canon Mathematicus, seu ad Triangula, cum Appendicibus*, and contains a great variety of tables useful in trigonometry. The first of these is what he more peculiarly calls *Canon Mathematicus, seu ad Triangula*, which contains all the sines, tangents, and secants for every minute of the quadrant, to the radius 100,000, with all their differences; and towards the end of the quadrant the tangents and secants are extended to 8 or 9 places of figures. They are arranged like our tables at present, increasing on the left hand side to 45 degrees, and then returning upwards by the right hand side to 90 degrees: so that each number and its complement stand on the same line. But here the canon of what we now call tangents is denominated *fœcundus*, and that of the secants *fœcundissimus*. For the general idea prevailing in the form of these tables, is, not that the lines represented by the numbers are those which are drawn in and about a circle, as sines, tangents, and secants, but the three sides of right-angled triangles; this being the way in which those lines had always been considered, and which still continued for some time longer. And therefore he considers the canon as a series of plane right-angled triangles, one side being constantly 100,000; or rather as three series of such triangles, for he makes a distinct series for each of the three varieties, namely, according as the hypotenuse, or the base, or the perpendicular, is represented by the constant number 100,000, which is similar to the radius. Making each side constantly 100,000, the other two sides are computed to every magnitude of the acute angle at the base, from 1 minute up to 90 degrees, or the whole quadrant. Each of the three series therefore consists of two parts, as representing the two variable sides of the triangle. When the hypotenuse is made the constant number 100,000, the two variable sides of the triangle are the perpendicular and base, or our sine and cosine; when the base is 100,000, the perpendicular and hypotenuse are the variable parts, forming the *canon fœcundus et fœcundissimus*, or our tangent and secant; and when the perpendicular is made the constant 100,000, the series contains the variable base and hypotenuse, or also *canon fœcundus et fœcundissimus*, or our cotangent and cosecant. Of course, therefore, the table consists of 6 columns, 2 for each of the 3 series, besides the two columns on the right and left for minutes, from 0 to 60 in each degree.

The second of these tables is similar to the first, but all in rational numbers, consisting, like *it*, of 3 series of 2 columns each; the radius, or constant side of the triangle, in each series, being 100,000, as before; and the other two sides *accurately* expressed in integers and rational vulgar fractions. So that we have here the canon of *accurate* sines, tangents, and secants; or a series of about 4300 rational right-angled triangles. But then the several corresponding arcs of the quadrant, or angles of those triangles, are not expressed. Instead of them, are inserted, in the first column next the margin, a series of numbers decreasing from the beginning to the end of the quadrant, which are called *numeri primi baseos*. It is from these numbers that Vieta constructs the sides of the 3 series of right-angled triangles, one side in each series being the constant number 100,000, as before. The theorems by which these series of rational triangles are computed from the *numeri primi baseos*, or marginal numbers, are inserted all in one page at the end of this second table, and in the modern notation they may be briefly expressed thus. Let p be the primary or marginal number on any line, and r the constant radius or number 100,000; then if r denote the hypotenuse of the right-angled triangle, the perpendicular and base, or the sine and cosine, will be respectively,

$$\frac{pr}{\frac{1}{2}p^2+1} \text{ and } r - \frac{2r}{\frac{1}{2}p^2+1}, \text{ (which last we may reduce to } \frac{\frac{1}{2}p^2-1}{\frac{1}{2}p^2+1}r\text{).}$$

When r denotes the base of the right-angled triangle, then the perpendicular and hypotenuse, or the tangent and secant, are expressed by
$\dfrac{pr}{\frac{1}{4}p^2-1}$ and $r+\dfrac{2r}{\frac{1}{4}p^2-1}$, (which last we may reduce to $\dfrac{\frac{1}{4}p^2+1}{\frac{1}{4}p^2-1}r$);
and when r denotes the perpendicular of the right-angled triangle, the base and hypotenuse, or the cotangent and cosecant, are then expressed by

$$\tfrac{1}{4}pr-\dfrac{r}{p}\ (\text{or}\ \dfrac{\frac{1}{4}p^2-1}{p}r),\ \text{and}\ \tfrac{1}{4}pr+\dfrac{r}{p}\ (\text{or}\ \dfrac{\frac{1}{4}p^2+1}{p}r).$$

So that Vieta's general values will be as we have here collected them together in the following expressions, immediately under the words sine, cosine, &c.; and just below Vieta's forms I have here placed the others to which they reduce and are equivalent, which are more contracted, though not so well adapted to the expeditious computation as Vieta's forms.

Sine	Cosine	Tangent	Secant	Cotangent	Cosecant
$\dfrac{pr}{\frac{1}{4}p^2+1}$	$r-\dfrac{2r}{\frac{1}{4}p^2+1}$	$\dfrac{pr}{\frac{1}{4}p^2-1}$	$r+\dfrac{2r}{\frac{1}{4}p^2-1}$	$\tfrac{1}{4}pr-\dfrac{r}{p}$	$\tfrac{1}{4}pr+\dfrac{r}{p}$
$\dfrac{p}{\frac{1}{4}p^2+1}r$	$\dfrac{\frac{1}{4}p^2-1}{\frac{1}{4}p^2+1}r$	$\dfrac{p}{\frac{1}{4}p^2-1}r$	$\dfrac{\frac{1}{4}p^2+1}{\frac{1}{4}p^2-1}r$	$\dfrac{\frac{1}{4}p^2-1}{p}r$	$\dfrac{\frac{1}{4}p^2+1}{p}r$

All these expressions, it is evident, are rational; and by assuming p of different values, from the first theorems Vieta computed the corresponding sides of the triangles, and so expressed them all in integers and rational fractions.

To the foregoing principal tables are subjoined several other smaller tables, or short specimens of large ones; as, a table of the sines, tangents, and secants for every single degree of the quadrant, with the corresponding lengths of the arcs, the radius being 100,000,000; another table of the sines, tangents, and secants, for each degree also, expressed in sexagesimal parts of the radius, as far as the 3d order of parts; also two other tables for the multiplication and reduction of sexagesimal quantities.

The second part of this volume is entitled *Universalium Inspectionum ad Canonem Mathematicum Liber singularis*. It contains the construction of the tables, a compendious treatise on plane and spherical trigonometry, with the application of them to a great variety of curious subjects in geometry and mensuration, treated in a very learned manner; as also many curious observations concerning the quadrature of the circle, the duplication of the cube, &c. Computations are here given of the ratio of the diameter of a circle to the circumference, and of the length of the sine of 1 minute, both to many places of figures; by which he found that the sine of 1 minute is between 2,908,881,959 and 2,908,882,056; also, the diameter of a circle being 1000, &c. that the perimeter of the inscribed and circumscribed polygon of 393216 sides, will be as follows:

perim. of the inscrib. polygon 314,159,265,35
perim. of the circum. polygon 314,159,265,37

and that therefore the circumference of the circle lies between those two numbers.

Though no author's name appears to the volume I have been describing, there can be no doubt of its being the performance of Vieta; for, besides bearing evident marks of his masterly hand, it is mentioned by himself in several parts of his other works collected by Schooten, and in the preface to those works by Elzevir the printer of them: as also in M. Montucla's *Histoire des Mathématiques*, which are the only notices I have ever seen or heard of concerning this book, the copies of which are so rare, that I never saw one besides that which is in my own possession.

In the other works of Vieta, published at Leyden in 1646, by Schooten, as mentioned above, there are several other pieces relating to trigonometry; some of which, on account of their originality and importance, are very deserving of particular notice in this place. And first, the very excellent theorems, here first of all given by our author, relating to angular sections, the geometrical demonstrations of which are supplied by that ingenious geometrician, Alexander Anderson, then professor of mathematics at Paris, but a native of Aberdeen, and cousin-german to Mr. David Anderson, of Finzaugh, whose daughter was the mother of the celebrated James Gregory, inventor of the Gregorian telescope. We find here, theorems of the chords (and consequently sines) of the sums and differences of arcs; and for the chords of arcs that are in arithmetical progression, namely, that the first or least chord is to the 2d, as any one after the 1st, is to the sum of the two next less and greater: for example, as the 2d to the sum of the 1st and 3d, and as the 3d to the sum of the 2d and 4th, and as the 4th to the sum of the 3d and 5th, &c.; so that, the 1st and 2d being given, all the rest are found from them by one subtraction and one proportion for each, in which the 1st and 2d terms are constantly the same. Next are given theorems for the chords of any multiples of a given arc or angle, as also the chords of their supplements to a semicircle, which are similar to the sines and cosines of the multiples of given angles; and the conclusions from them are expressed in this manner; 1st, that if c be the chord of the supplement of a given arc a, to the radius 1, then the chords of the supplements of the multiple arcs will be as in the annexed table: where the author observes that the signs are alternately $+$ and $-$; that the vertical columns of numeral coefficients to the terms of the chords, are the several orders of figurate numbers, which he calls triangular, pyramidal, triangulo-triangular, triangulo-pyramidal, &c. *generated in the ordinary way by continual additions; not indeed from unity, AS IN THE GENERATION OF POWERS, but beginning with the number 2; and*

Arcs	Chords of the Supplements.
1a	c
2a	$c^2 - 2$
3a	$c^3 - 3c$
4a	$c^4 - 4c^2 + 2$
5a	$c^5 - 5c^3 + 5c$
6a	$c^6 - 6c^4 + 9c^2 - 2$
7a	$c^7 - 7c^5 + 14c^3 - 7c$
&c.	&c.

positions, the construction of the canon to the radius 10000000000000000. By some of the common properties of geometry, having determined the sines of a few principal arcs, as 30°, 36°, &c. in the first proposition, by continual bisections he finds the sines of various other arcs, down to 45 minutes. Then in the 2d proposition, by the theorems for the sums and differences of arcs, he finds all the sines and cosines, up to 90 degrees, in a series of arcs differing by 1° 30'. And, in the 3d proposition, by the continual addition of 45', he obtains all the sines and cosines in the series whose common difference is 45'. In the 4th proposition, beginning with 45', and continually bisecting, he finds the sines and cosines of the series of half arcs, till he arrives at the arc of 14^{viii} 19^{ix}, the sine of which is found to be 1, and its cosine 999999999999999. In the fifth proposition are computed the sine and cosine of 30'', or half a minute. In the 6th and 7th propositions are computed the sines and cosines for every minute, from 1' to 45', as well as of many larger arcs. The 8th proposition extends the computation for single minutes much further. In propositions 9 and 10 are computed the tangents and secants for all arcs in the series whose common difference is 45'; and these are deduced from the sines of the same arcs by one proportion for each. In the remaining three propositions, 11, 12, 13, are computed the tangents and secants for several small angles. And from all these primary sines, tangents, and secants, the whole canon is deduced and completed.

The remaining books in this work are by the editor Otho; namely, a treatise, in one book, on right-angled plane triangles, the cases of which are resolved by the tables: then right-angled spherical trigonometry, in four books; next oblique spherical trigonometry, in five books; and lastly, several other books, containing various spherical problems.

Next after the above are placed the tables themselves, containing the sines, tangents, and secants, for every 10 seconds in the quadrant, with all the differences annexed to each, in a smaller character. The numbers however are not called sines, tangents, and secants, but, like Vieta's before described, they are considered as representing the sides of right-angled triangles, and titled accordingly. They are also, in like manner, divided into three series, namely, according as the radius, or constant side of the triangle, is made the hypotenuse, or the greater leg, or the less leg of the triangle. When the hypotenuse is made the constant radius 10000000000, the two columns of this case, or series, are called the perpendicular and base, which are our sine and cosine; when the greater leg is the constant radius, the two columns of this series are titled hypotenuse and perpendicular, which are our secant and tangent; and when the less leg is constant, the two columns in this case are called hypotenuse and base, which are our cosecant and cotangent. After this large canon, is printed another smaller table, which is said to be the two columns of the third series, or cosecants and cotangents, with their differences, but to 3 places of figures less, or to the radius 10000000. But I cannot discover the reason for adding this less table, even if it were correct, which is very far from being the case, the numbers being uniformly erroneous, and different from the former through the greatest part of the table.

Towards the close of the 16th century, many persons wrote on the subject of trigonometry, and the construction of the triangular canon. But, their writings being seldom printed till many years afterwards, it is not easy to assign their order in respect of time. I shall therefore mention but a few of the principal authors, and that without pretending to any great precision on the score of chronological precedence.

In 1591 Philip Lansberg first published his *Geometria Triangulorum*, in four books, with the canon of sines, tangents, and secants; a brief, but very elegant work; the whole being clearly explained: and it is perhaps the first set of tables titled with those words. The sines, tangents and secants of the arcs to 45· degrees, with those of their complements, are each placed in adjacent columns, in a very commodious manner, continued forwards and downwards to 45 degrees, and then returning backwards and upwards to 90 degrees: the radius is 10000000, and a specimen of the first page of the table is as follows:

0	Sinus		Tangens		Secans		
0	0	10000000	0	infinitum.	10000000	infinitum.	60
1	2909	9999999	2909	34377466738	10000002	34377468193	59
2	5818	9999998	5818	17188731915	10000004	17188734924	58
3	8727	9999996	8727	11459152994	10000004	11459157357	57
4	11636	9999993	11636	8594363048	10000007	8594368866	56
5	14544	9999989	14544	6875488693	10000011	6875495966	55
&c.							&c.
							89

Of this work, the first book treats of the magnitude and relations of such lines as are considered in and about the circle, as the chords, sines, tangents, and secants. In the second book is delivered the construction of the trigonometrical canon, by means of the properties laid down in the first book. After which follows the canon itself. And in the third and fourth books is shown the application of the table, in the resolution of plane and spherical triangles——Lansberg, who was born in Zealand 1561, was many years a minister of the gospel, and died at Middleburg in 1632.

The trigonometry of Bartholomew Pitiscus was first published at Francfort in the year 1599. This is a very complete work; containing, besides the triangular canon, with its construction and use in resolving triangles, the application of trigonometry to problems of surveying, altimetry, architecture, geography, dialling, and astronomy. The construction of the canon is very clearly described: And, in the third edition of the book, in the year 1612, he boasts to have added in this part arithmetical rules for finding the chords of the 3d, 5th, and other uneven parts of an arc, from the chord of that arc being given; saying, that it had been heretofore thought impossible to give such rules: But, after all, those boasted methods are only the application of the double rule of False-Position to the then known rules for finding the chords of multiple arcs; namely, making the supposition of some number for the required chord of a submultiple of any given arc, then, from this assumed number, computing what will be the chord of its multiple arc; which is to be compared with that of the given arc; then the same operation is performed with another supposition, and so on, as in the double rule of position. The canon contains the sine, tangent, and secant, for every minute of the quadrant, in some parts to 7 places of figures, in others to 8; as also the differences for every 10 seconds. The sines, tangents, and secants, are also given for every 10 seconds in the first and last degree of the quadrant, for every 2 seconds in the first and last 10 minutes, and for every single second in the first and last minute. In this table the sines, tangents, and secants are continued downwards on the left-hand pages as far as to 45 degrees, and then returned upwards on the right-hand pages, so that the complements are always on the same line in the opposite or facing pages.

The mathematical works of Christopher Clavius (a German jesuit, who was born at Bamberg in 1537) in five large folio volumes, were printed at Moguntia, or Mentz, in 1612, the year in which the author died, at the age of 75. In the first volume we find a very ample and circumstantial treatise on trigonometry, with Regiomontanus's canon of sines, for every minute, as also canons of tangents and secants, each in a separate table, to the radius 10000000, and in a form continued forwards all the way up to 90 degrees. The explanation of the construction of the tables is very complete, and is chiefly extracted from Ptolemy, Purbach, and Regiomontanus. The sines have the differences set down for each second, that is, the quotients arising from the differences of the sines divided by 60.

About the year 1600, Ludolph van Collen, or à Ceulen, a respectable Dutch mathematician, wrote his book *De Circulo et Adscriptis*, in which he treats fully and ably of the properties of lines drawn in and about the circle, and especially of chords or subtenses, with the construction of the canon of sines. The geometrical properties from which these lines are computed, are the same as those used by former writers; but his mode of computing and expressing them is different from theirs; for they actually extracted all the roots, &c, at every step, or single operation, in decimal numbers; but he retained the radical expressions to the last, making them however always as simple as possible: thus, for instance, he determines the sides of the polygons of 4, 8, 16, 32, &c, sides, inscribed in the circle whose radius is 1, to be as in the table here annexed: where the point before any figure (as $\sqrt{.2}$) signifies the root of all that follows it; so the last line is in our notation the same as

$$\sqrt{.2-\sqrt{.2+\sqrt{.2-\sqrt{.2}}}}.$$ And as the perfect management of such surds was then not generally

No. of sides.	Length of each side.
4	$\sqrt{.2}$
8	$\sqrt{.2-\sqrt{.2}}$
16	$\sqrt{.2-\sqrt{.2+\sqrt{.2}}}$
32	$\sqrt{.2-\sqrt{.2+\sqrt{.2-\sqrt{.2}}}}$
&c.	&c.

known, he added a very neat tract on that subject, to facilitate the computations. These, together with other dissertations on similar geometrical matters, were translated from the Dutch language, into Latin, by Willebrord Snell, and published at (Lugd. Batav.) Leyden in 1619. It was in this work that Ludolph determined the ratio of the diameter to the circumference of the circle, to 36 figures, showing that, if the diameter be 1, the circumference will be

greater than 3.14159 26535 89793 23846 26433 83279 50288,

but less than 3.14159 26535 89793 23846 26433 83279 50289; which ratio was, by his order, in imitation of Archimedes, engraven on his tomb-stone, as is witnessed by the said Snell, pa. 54, 55, *Cyclometricus*, published at Leyden two years after, in which he treats the same subject in a similar manner, recomputing and verifying Ludolph's numbers. And in the same book, he also gives a variety of geometrical approximations, or mechanical solutions, to determine very nearly the lengths of arcs, and the areas of sectors and segments of circles.

Besides the *Cyclometricus*, and another geometrical work (*Apollonius Battavus*) published in 1608, the same Snellius wrote also four others, *doctrinæ triangulorum canonicæ*, in which is contained the canon of secants, and in which the construction of sines, tangents, and secants, together with the dimension or calculation of triangles, both plane and spherical, are briefly and clearly treated. After the author's death, this work was published in 8vo, at Leyden 1627, by Martinus Hortensius, who added to it a tract on surveying and spherical problems. Willebrord Snell was born in 1591 at Royen, and died in 1626, being only 35 years of age. He was professor of mathematics in the university of Leyden, as was also his father Rodolph Snell.

In 1627, Francis van Schooten published, at Amsterdam, in a small neat form, tables of sines, tangents, and secants, for every minute of the quadrant, to 7 places of figures, the radius being 10000000; together with their use in plane trigonometry. These tables have a great character for their accuracy, being declared by the author to be without one single error. This however must not be understood of the last figure of the numbers, which I find are very often erroneous, sometimes in excess and sometimes in defect, by not being always set down to the nearest unit. Schooten died in 1659, while he had the second volume of his second edition of Descartes' geometry in the press. He was also author of several other valuable works in geometry and other branches of the mathematics.

The foregoing are the principal writers on the tables of sines, tangents, and secants, before the invention of logarithms, which happened about this time, namely, soon after the year 1600. Tables of the natural numbers were now all completed, and the methods of computing them nearly perfected: And therefore, before entering on the discovery and construction of logarithms, we shall stop here a little, to give a summary of the manner in which the said natural sines, tangents, and secants, were actually computed, after having been gradually improved from Hipparchus, Menelaus, and Ptolemy, who used only the chords, down to the beginning of the 17th century, when sines, tangents, secants, and versed sines were in use, and when the method hitherto employed had received its utmost improvement. In this explanation, I shall here first enumerate the theorems by which the calculations were made, and then describe the application of them to the computation itself.

Theorem 1. The square of the diameter of a circle, is equal to the sum of the squares of the chord of an arc, and of the chord of its supplement to a semicircle.

2. The rectangle under the two diagonals of any quadrilateral inscribed in a circle, is equal to the sum of the two rectangles under the opposite sides.

3. The sum of the squares of the sine and cosine (hitherto called the sine of the complement), is equal to the square of the radius.

4. The difference between the sines of two arcs that are equally distant from 60 degrees, or $\frac{1}{6}$ of the whole circumference, the one as much greater as the other is less, is equal to the sine of half the differences of those arcs, or of the difference between either arc and the said arc of 60 degrees.

5. The sum of the cosine and versed sine, is equal to the radius.

6. The sum of the squares of the sine and versed sine, is equal to the square of the chord, or to the square of double the sine of half the arc.

7. The sine is a mean proportional between half the radius and the versed sine of double the arc.

8. A mean proportional between the versed sine and half the radius, is equal to the sine of half the arc.

9. As radius is to the sine, so is twice the cosine to the sine of twice the arc.

10. As the chord of an arc, is to the sum of the chords of the single and double arc, so is the difference of those chords, to the chord of thrice the arc.

11. As the chord of an arc, is to the sum of the chords of twice and thrice the arc, so is the difference of those chords, to the chord of five times the arc.

12. And in general, as the chord of an arc, is to the sum of the chords of n times and $n+1$ times the arc, so is the difference of those chords, to the chord of $2n+1$ times the arc.

13. The sine of the sum of two arcs, is equal to the sum of the products of the sine of each multiplied by the cosine of the other, and divided by the radius.

14. The sine of the difference of two arcs, is equal to the difference of the said two products divided by radius.

15. The cosine of the sum of two arcs, is equal to the difference between the products of their sines and of their cosines, divided by radius.

16. The cosine of the difference of two arcs, is equal to the sum of the said products divided by radius.

17. A small arc is equal to its chord or sine, nearly.

18. As cosine is to sine, so is radius to tangent.

19. Radius is a mean proportional between the tangent and co-tangent.

20. Half the difference between the tangent and cotangent of an arc, is equal to the tangent of the difference between the arc and its complement. Or, the sum arising from the addition of double the tangent of an arc with the tangent of half its complement, is equal to the tangent of the sum of that arc and the said half complement.

21. The square of the secant of an arc, is equal to the sum of the squares of the radius and tangent.

22. Radius is a mean proportional between the secant and cosine. Or, as cosine is to radius, so is radius to secant.

23. Radius is a mean proportional between the sine and cosecant.

24. The secant of an arc, is equal to the sum of its tangent and the tangent of half its complement. Or, the secant of the difference between an arc and its complement, is equal to the tangent of the said difference added to the tangent of the less arc.

25. The secant of an arc, is equal to the difference between the tangent of that arc and the tangent of the arc added to half its complement. Or the secant of the difference between an arc and its complement, is equal to the difference between the tangent of the said difference and the tangent of the greater arc.

From some of these 25 theorems, extracted from the writers before mentioned, and a few propositions of Euclid's elements, they compiled the whole table of sines, tangents, and secants, nearly in the following manner. By the elements were computed the sides of a few of the regular figures inscribed in a circle, which were the chords of such parts of the whole circumference as are expressed by the number of sides, and therefore the halves of those chords the sines of the halves of the arcs. So, if the radius be 10000000, the sides of the following figures will give the annexed chords and sines.

The figure	Arc sub-tended	Its chord, or side	Half arc	Its sine, or ½ chord
Triangle	120°	17320508	60°	8660254
Square	90	14142136	45	7071068
Pentagon	72	11755705	36	5877853
Hexagon	60	10000000	30	5000000
Decagon	36	6180340	18	3090170
Quindecagon	24	4158234	12	2079117

Of some, or all of these, the sines of the halves were continually taken by theorem the 6th, 7th, or 8th, and of their complements by the 3d; then the sines of the halves of these, and of their complements, by the same theorems; and so on, alternately of the halves and complements, till they arrived at an arc which is nearly equal to its sine. Thus, beginning with the above arc of 12 degrees, and its sine, the halves were obtained as follows:

The halves		Their Sines
6°	′	1045285
3		523360
1	30	261769
.	45	130896
The comp. of these		
84		9945218
87		9986295
88	30	9996573
89	15	9999143
The halves of these		
42		6691306
21		3583679
10	30	1822355
5	15	915016
43	30	6883545
21	45	3705574
44	15	6977905

The Comp. of these		Sines
48°	′	7431448
69		9335804
79	30	9832549
84	45	9958049
46	30	7253744
68	15	9288095
45	45	7163019
The halves of these		
24		4067366
34	30	5664062
17	15	2965416
39	45	6394390
23	15	3947439
The comp.		
66		9135455
55	30	8241262
72	45	9550199
50	15	7688418
66	45	9187912

The halves		Sines
33°	′	5446390
16	30	2840153
8	15	1434926
27	45	4656145
Comps.		
57		8386706
73	30	9588197
81	45	9896514
62	15	8849876
Halves		
28	30	4771588
14	15	2461533
36	45	5983246
Comps.		
61	30	8788171
75	45	9692309
53	15	8012538
Half		
30	45	5112931
Comp.		
59	15	8594064

The sines of small arcs are then deduced in this manner: From the sine of 45′, above determined, are found the halves, which will be thus :

$$
\begin{array}{llll}
45′ & 0″ & \ldots\ldots & 130896 \\
22 & 30 & \ldots\ldots & 65449,4 \\
11 & 15 & \ldots\ldots & 32724,8
\end{array}
$$

Now these last two sines being evidently in the same ratio as their arcs, the sines of all the less single minutes will be found by single proportion. So the 45th part of the sine of 45′, gives 2909 for the sine of 1′; which may be doubled, tripled, &c, for the sines of 2′, 3′, &c, up to 45′.

Then, from all the foregoing primary sines, by the theorems for halving, doubling, or tripling, and by those for the sums and differences, the rest of the sines are deduced, to complete the quadrant.

But having thus determined the sines and cosines of the first 30° of the quadrant, that is, the sines of the first and last 30°, those of the intermediate 30° are, by theor. 4, found by one single subtraction for each sine.

The sines of the whole quadrant being thus completed, the tangents are found by theor. 18, 19, 20, namely, for one half of the quadrant by the 18th and 19th, and the other half by one single addition or subtraction for each, by the 20th theorem.

And lastly by theor. 24 and 25, the secants are deduced from the tangents, by addition and subtraction only.

Among the various means used for constructing the canon of sines, tangents, and secants, the writers above enumerated seem not to have been possessed of the method of differences, so profitably used since, and first of all I believe by Briggs, in computing his trigonometrical canon and his logarithms, as we shall see hereafter, when we come to describe those works. They took however the successive differences of the numbers after they were computed, to verify or prove the truth of them; and if found erroneous, by any irregularity in the last differences, from thence they had a method of correcting the original numbers themselves. At least, this method is used by Pitiscus, *Trig. lib.* 2, where the differences are extended to the third order.——In page 44 of the same book also is described, for the first time that I know of, the common notation of decimal fractions, as now used. And this same notation was afterwards described and used by baron Napier, in *positio* 4 and 5 of his posthumous works, on the construction of logarithms, published by his son in the year 1619. But the decimal fractions themselves may be considered as having been introduced by Regiomontanus, by his decimal division of the radius &c, of the circle; and from that time gradually brought into use: but continued long to be denoted after the manner of vulgar fractions, by a line drawn between the numerator and denominator, which last however was soon omitted, and only the numerator set down, with the line below it; thus it was first $31\frac{35}{100}$, then $31\overset{35}{}$; afterwards, omitting the line, it became 31^{35}, and lastly 31_{35}, or 31.35, or 31·35: as may be traced in the works of Vieta, and others since his time, gradually into the present century.

Having often heard it remarked, that the word *sine*, or in Latin and French *sinus*, is of doubtful origin; and as the various accounts which I have seen of its derivation are very different from one another, it may not be amiss here to employ a few lines on this matter. Some authors say, this is an Arabic word, others that it is the single Latin word *sinus*; and in Montucla's *Histoire des Mathematiques* it is conjectured to be an abbreviation of two Latin words*. The conjecture is thus expressed by the ingenious and learned author of that excellent history, at pa. xxxiii, among the additions and corrections of the first volume: " A l'occasion des sinus dont on parle dans cette page, comme d'une invention des Arabes, voici un étymologie de ce nom, tout-à-fait heureuse et vraisemblable. Je la dois à M. Godin, de l'Académie Royale des Sciences, Directeur de l'Ecole de Marine de Cadix. Les sinus sont, comme l'on sçait, des moitiés de cordes ; et les cordes en Latin se nomment *inscriptæ*. Les sinus sont donc *semisses inscriptarum*, ce que probablement on écrivit ainsi pour abréger, S. Ins. Delà ensuite s'est fait par abus le mot de sinus." Now, ingenious as this conjecture is, there appears to be little or no probability for the truth of it. For, in the first place, it is not in the least supported by quotations from any of the more early books, to show that it ever was the practice to write or print the words thus, *S. Ins.* on which the conjecture is founded. Again, it is said the chords are called in Latin *inscriptæ*; and it is true that they sometimes are so: but I think they are more frequently called *subtensæ*, and the sines *semisses subtensarum*

---

* That is, in the first edition of his book. But he has omitted this improbable conjecture in the new edition of 1799.

of the double arcs, which will not abbreviate into the word *sinus*.
But it may be said, what reason have we to suppose that this word is
either a Latin word, or the abbreviation of any Latin words whatever? and that it seems but proper to seek for the etymology of
words in the language of the inventors of the *things*. For which
reason it is, that we find the two other words, *tangens* and *secans*, are
Latin, as they were invented and used by authors who wrote in that
language. But the sines are acknowledged to have been invented
and introduced by the Arabians, and thence by analogy it would
seem probable that this is a word of *their* language, and from them
adopted, together with the use of it, by the Europeans. And indeed
Lansberg, in the second page of his trigonometry above mentioned,
expressly says that it *is* Arabic: His words are, *Vox sinus Arabica est,
et proinde bàrbara ; sed cùm longo usu approbata sit, et commodior non
suppetat, nequaquam repudianda est : faciles enim in verbis nos esse opor-
tet, cum de rebus convenit*. And Vieta says something to the same pur-
port, in page 9 of his *Universalium Inspectionum ad Canonem Mathematicum Liber:* His words are, *Breve sinus vocabulum, cùm sit artis,
Saracenis præsertim quàm familiare, non est ab artificibus exploden-
dum, ad laterum semissium inscriptorum denotationem, &c.*

Guarinus also is of the same opinion: in his *Euclides Adauctus, &c,*
tract. xx. pa. 307, he says, SINUS *verò est nomen Arabicum usurpatum in
hanc significationem à mathematicis ;* though he was aware that a Latin
origin was ascribed to it by Vitalis, for he immediately adds, *Licèt Vitalis in suo Lexico Mathematico ex eo velit sinum appellatum, quòd
claudat curvitatem arcús.*

Long before I either saw or heard of any conjecture, or observation
concerning the etymology of the word *sinus*, I remember that I *imagined* it to be taken from the same Latin word, signifying breast or bosom, and that our sine was so called allegorically. I had observed,
that several of the terms in trigonometry were derived from a bow to
shoot with, and its appendages; as *arcus*, the bow, *chorda*, the string,
and *sagitta*, the arrow, by which name the versed sine, which repre-
sents it, was sometimes called; also, that the *tangens* was so called
from its office, being a line *touching* the circle, and *secans* from its *cutting* the same: I therefore imagined that the *sinus* was so called, either
from its resemblance to the breast or bosom, or from its being a line
drawn within the bosom *(sinus)* of the arc, or from its being that part
of the string *(chorda)* of a bow *(arcus)* which is drawn near the
breast *(sinus)* in the act of shooting. And perhaps Vitalis's definition, above quoted, has some allusion to the same similitude.

Also Vieta seems to allude to the same thing, in calling *sinus* an
allegorical word, in page 417 of his works, as published by Schooten,
where, with his usual judgement and precision, he treats of the propriety of the terms used in trigonometry for certain lines drawn in
and about the circle; of which, as it very well deserves, I shall here
extract the principal part, to show the opinion and arguments of so
great a man on those names. " *Arabes autem semisses inscriptas du-
plo, numeris præsertim æstimatas, vocaverunt allegoricè* SINUS, *atque
ideo ipsam semi-diametrum, quæ maxima est semissium inscriptarum,*
SINUM TOTUM. *Et de iis suâ methodo canones exiverunt qui circum-*

feruntur, supputante præsertim Regiomontano benè justè et accuratè, in iis etiam particulis qualium semidiameter adsumitur 10,000,000.

" Ex canonibus deinde sinuum derivaverunt recentiores canonem semissium circumscriptarum, quem dixêre *Fœcundum*; et canonem eductarum è centro, quem dixêre *Fœcundissimum* et *Beneficum*, hypotenusis addictum. Atque adeò semisses circumscriptas, numeris præsertim æstimatas, vocaverunt *Fœcundos*, Sinus numeròsve videlicet; quanquam nihil vetat *Fœcundi* nomen substantivè accipi. Hypotenusas autem Beneficas, yel etiam simpliciter Hypotenusas: quoniam hypotenusa in primâ serie sinûs totius nomen retinet. Itaque ne novitate verborum res adumbretur, et alioqui sua artificibus, eo nomine debita, præripiatur gloria, præposita in Canone Mathematico canonicis numeris inscriptio, candidè admonet primam seriem esse Canonem Sinuum. In secundâ verò, partem canonis fœcundi, partem canonis fœcundissimi, contineri. In tertiâ, reliquam.

" Sanè præter inscriptas et circumscriptas, circulum etiam adficiunt aliæ lineæ rectæ, velut Incidentes, Tangentes, et Secantes. Verùm illæ voces substantivæ sunt, non peripheriarum relativæ. Ac secare quidem circulum linea recta tunc intelligitur, cùm in duobus punctis secat. Itaque non loquuntur benè geometricè, qui eductas è centro ad metas circumscriptarum vocant secantes impropriè, cum secantes et tangentes ad certos angulos vel peripherias referunt. Immò verò artem confundunt, cùm his vocibus necesse habeat uti geometra abs relatione.

" Quare si quibus arrideat Arabum metaphora; quæ quidem aut omninò retinenda videtur, aut omninò explodenda; ut semisses inscriptas, Arabes vocant sinus; sic semisses circumscriptæ, vocentur Prosinus Amsinusve; et eductæ è centro Transsinuosæ. Sin allegoria displiceat, geometrica sane inscriptarum et circumscriptarum nomina retineantur. Et cùm eductæ è centro ad metas circumscriptarum, non habeant hactenus nomen certum neque elegans, vocentur sanè prosemidiametri, quasi protensæ semidiametri, se habentes ad suas circumscriptas, sicut semidiametri ad inscriptas."

Against the Arabic origin however of this word *(sinus)* may be urged its being varied according to the fourth declension of Latin nouns like *manus*; and that if it were an Arabic word latinised, it would have been ranked under either the first, second, or third declension, as is usual in such adopted words.

So that, upon the whole, it will perhaps rather seem probable, that the term *sinus* is the Latin word answering to the name by which the Saracens called that line, and not their word itself. And this conjecture seems to be rendered still more probable by some expressions in pa. 4 and 5 of Otho's Preface to Rheticus's Canon, where it is not only said, that the Saracens called the half-chord of double the arc *sinus*, but also that they called the part of the radius lying between the sine and the arc *sinus versus, vel sagitta*, which are evidently Latin words, and seem to be intended for the Latin translations of the names by which the Arabians called these lines, or the numbers expressing the lengths of them.

And this conjecture has been confirmed and realised, by a reference to Golius's Lexicon of the Arabic and Latin languages. In consequence I find that the Arabic and Latin writers on trigonometry do both of them use those words in the same allegorical sense, the latter being

D 2

the Latin translations of the former, and not the Arabic words corrupted. Thus the true Arabic word to denote the trigonometrical sine, is جيـب, pronounced *Jeib* (reading the vowels in the French manner), meaning *sinus indusii, vestisque*, the bosom part of the garment : the versed sine is سهـم, *Sehim*, which is *sagitta*, the arrow; the arc is قــر س, which is *arcus*, the arc; and the chord is وتـر, *Vitr*, that is, *chorda*, the chord.

OF LOGARITHMS.

THE trigonometrical canon of natural sines, tangents and secants, being now brought to a considerable degree of perfection, the great length and accuracy of the numbers, together with the increasing delicacy and number of astronomical problems and spherical triangles, to the solution of which the canon was applied, urged many persons, conversant in those matters, to endeavour to discover some means of diminishing the great labour and time, requisite for so many multiplications and divisions, in such large numbers as the tables then consisted of. And their chief aim was, to reduce the multiplications and divisions to additions and subtractions, as much as possible.

For this purpose, Nicholas Raymer Ursus Dithmarsus invented an ingenious method, which serves for one case in the sines, namely, when radius is the first term in the proportion, and the sines of two arcs are the second and third terms; for he showed, that the fourth term, or sine, would be found by only taking half the sum or difference of the sines of two other arcs, which should be the sum and difference of the less of the two former given arcs, and the complement of the greater. This is no more, in effect, than the following well-known theorem in trigonometry : as half radius is to the sine of one arc, so is the sine of another arc, to the cosine of the difference *minus* the cosine of the sum of the said arcs. The author published this ingenious device in 1588, in his *Fundamentum Astronomiæ*. And three or four years afterwards it was greatly improved by Clavius, who adapted it to all proportions in the resolution of the spherical triangles, for all sines, tangents, secants, versed sines, &c; and that whether radius be in the proportion or not. All which he explains very fully in *lem.* 53, *lib.* 1, of his treatise on the *Astrolabe*. See more on this subject in Longomont. Astron. Danica, pa. 7, et seq. This method, though ingenious, depends not on any abstract property of numbers, but only on the relations of certain lines, drawn in and about the circle ; and it was therefore rather limited, and sometimes attended with trouble in the application.

After perhaps various other contrivances, incessant endeavours at length produced the happy invention of logarithms, which are of direct and universal application to all numbers abstractedly considered, being derived from a property inherent in numbers themselves. This property may be considered, either as the relation between a geometrical series of terms and a corresponding arithmetical one, or as the relation between ratios and the measures of ratios, which comes to much the same thing, having been conceived in one of these ways by some of the writers on this subject, and in the other by the rest of them, as well as in both ways at different times by the same writer. A succinct idea of this property, and of the probable reflections made on it by the first writers on logarithms, may be to the following effect:

The learned calculators, about the close of the 16th, and beginning of the 17th century, finding the operations of multiplication and division by very long numbers, of seven or eight places of figures, which they had frequently occasion to perform, in resolving problems relating to geography and astronomy, to be exceedingly troublesome, set themselves to consider whether it was not possible to find some method of lessening this labour, by substituting other easier operations in their stead. In pursuit of this object, they reflected, that, since, in every multiplication by a whole number, the ratio, or proportion, of the product to the multiplicand, is the same as the ratio of the multiplier to unity, it will follow that the ratio of the product to unity (which, according to Euclid's definition of compound ratios, is compounded of the ratios of the said product to the multiplicand and of the multiplicand to unity), must be equal to the sum of the two ratios of the multiplier to unity and of the multiplicand to unity. Consequently, if they could find a set of artificial numbers that should be the representatives of, or should be proportional to, the ratios of all sorts of numbers to unity, the addition of the two artificial numbers that should represent the ratios of any multiplier and multiplicand to unity, would answer to the multiplication of the said multiplicand by the said multiplier, or the sum arising from the addition of the said representative numbers would be the representative number of the ratio of the product to unity; and consequently, the natural number to which it should be found, in the table of the said artificial or representative numbers, that the said sum belonged, would be the product of the said multiplicand and multiplier. Having settled this principle, as the foundation of their wished-for method of abridging the labour of calculations, they resolved to compose a table of such artificial numbers, or numbers that should be representatives of, or proportional to, the ratios of all the common or natural numbers to unity.

The first observation that naturally occurred to them in the pursuit of this scheme, was, that whatever artificial numbers should be chosen to represent the ratios of other whole numbers to unity, the ratio of equality, or of unity to unity, must be represented by 0; because *that* ratio has properly no magnitude, since, when it is added to, or subtracted from, any other ratio, it neither increases nor diminishes it.

The second observation that occurred to them was, that any number whatever might be chosen at pleasure for the representative of the ratio of any given natural number to unity; but that, when once such choice was made, all the other representative numbers would be thereby determined, because they must be greater or less than that first representative number, in the same proportions in which the ratios represented by them, or the ratios of the corresponding natural numbers to unity, were greater or less than the ratio of the said given natural number to unity. Thus, either 1, or 2, or 3, &c, might be chosen for the representative of the ratio of 10 to 1. But, if 1 be chosen for it, the representative of the ratio of 100 to 1 and 1000 to 1, which are double and triple of the ratio of 10 to 1, must be 2 and 3, and cannot be any other numbers: and if 2 be chosen for it, then the representatives of the ratios of 100 to 1 and 1000 to 1, will be 4 and 6, and cannot be any other numbers; and if 3 be chosen for it, then the representatives of the ratios of 100 to 1 and 1000 to 1, will be 6 and 9, and cannot be any other numbers; and so on.

The third observation that occurred to them was, that, as these artificial numbers were representatives of, or proportional to, ratios of the natural numbers to unity, they must be expressions of the numbers of some smaller equal ratios that are contained in the said ratios. Thus, if 1 be taken for the representative of the ratio of 10 to 1, then 3, which is the representative of the ratio of 1000 to 1, will express the number of ratios of 10 to 1 that are contained in the ratio of 1000 to 1. And if, instead of 1, we make 10,000,000, or ten millions, the representative of the ratio of 10 to 1 (in which case 1 will be the representative of a very small ratio, or *ratiuncula*, which is only the ten-millionth part of the ratio of 10 to 1, or will be the representative of the 10,000,000th root of 10, or of the first or smallest of 9,999,999 mean proportionals interposed between 1 and 10), the representative of the ratio of 1000 to 1, which will in this case be 30,000,000, will express the number of those *ratiuncula*, or small ratios of the 10,000,000th root of 10 to 1, which are contained in the said ratio of 1000 to 1. And the like may be shown of the representative of the ratio of any other number to unity. And therefore they thought these artificial numbers, which thus represent, or are proportional to, the magnitudes of the ratios of the natural numbers to unity, might not improperly be called the LOGARITHMS of those ratios, since they express the numbers of smaller ratios of which they are composed. And then, for the sake of brevity, they called them the *Logarithms of the said natural numbers themselves*, which are the antecedents of the said ratios to unity, of which they are in truth the representatives.

The foregoing method of considering this property leads to much the same conclusions as the other way, in which the relations between a geometrical series of terms, and their exponents, or the terms of an arithmetical series, are contemplated. In this latter way, it readily occurred that the addition of the terms of the arithmetical series corresponded to the multiplication of the terms of the geometrical series; and that the arithmeticals would therefore form a set of artificial numbers, which, when arranged in tables, with their geometricals, would answer the purposes desired, as has been explained above.

From this property, by assuming four quantities, two of them as two terms in a geometrical series, and the others as the two corresponding terms of the arithmeticals, or artificials, or logarithms, it is evident that all the other terms of both the two series may thence be generated. And therefore there may be as many sets or scales of logarithms as we please, since they depend entirely on the arbitrary assumption of the first two arithmeticals. And all possible natural numbers may be supposed to coincide with some of the terms of any geometrical progression whatever, the logarithms or arithmeticals determining which of the terms in that progression they are.

It was proper however that the arithmetical series should be so as-

sumed, as that the term 0 in it might answer to the term 1 in the geometricals; otherwise the sum of the logarithms of any two numbers
would be always to be diminished by the logarithm of 1, to give the
logarithm of the product of those numbers: for which reason, making
0 the logarithm of 1, and assuming any quantity whatever for the value
of the logarithm of any one number, the logarithms of all other numbers were thence to be derived. And hence, like as the multiplication
of two numbers is effected by barely adding their logarithms, so division is performed by subtracting the logarithm of the one from that
of the other, raising of powers by multiplying the logarithm of the
given number by the index of the power, and extraction of roots by
dividing the logarithm by the index of the root. It is also evident, that
in all scales or systems of logarithms, the logarithm of 0 will be infinite;
namely, infinitely negative if the logarithms increase with the natural
numbers, but infinitely positive if the contrary; because that while the
geometrical series must decrease through infinite divisions by the ratio
of the progression, before the quotient come to 0 or nothing; the logarithms, or arithmeticals, will in like manner undergo the corresponding infinite subtractions or additions of the common equal difference;
which equal increase or decrease, thus indefinitely continued, must
needs tend to an infinite result.

This however was no newly-discovered property of numbers, but
what was always well known to all mathematicians, being treated of
in the writings of Euclid, as also by Archimedes, who made great
use of it in his *Arenarius*, or treatise on the number of the sands,
namely, in assigning the rank or place of those terms, of a geometrical
series produced from the multiplication together of any of the foregoing terms, by the addition of the corresponding terms of the arithmetical series, which served as the indices or exponents of the former.
Stifelius also treats very fully of this property at folio 35 et seq. and
there explains all its principal uses, as relating to the logarithms of
numbers, only without the name; such as, that addition answers to
multiplication, subtraction to division, multiplication of exponents to
involution, and dividing of exponents to evolution; all which he exemplifies in the rule-of-three, and in finding several mean proportionals, &c, exactly as is done in logarithms. So that he seems to have
been in the full possession of the idea of logarithms, but without the
necessity of making a table of such numbers. For, the reason why
tables of these numbers were not sooner composed, was, that the accuracy and trouble of trigonometrical computations had not sooner
rendered them necessary. It is therefore not to be doubted, that
about the close of the sixteenth and beginning of the seventeenth
century, many persons had thoughts of such a table of numbers, besides the few who are said to have attempted it.

It has been said by some, that Longomontanus invented logarithms:
but this cannot well be supposed to have been any more than in idea,
since he never published any thing of the kind, nor ever laid claim to
the invention, though he lived thirty-three years after they were first

published by baron Napier, as he died only in 1647, when they had been long known and received all over Europe. Nay more, Longomontanus himself ascribes the invention to Napier: vid. Astron. Danica, p. 7, &c. Some circumstances of this matter are indeed related by Wood in his *Athenæ Oxonienses*, under the article Briggs, on the authority of Oughtred and Wingate, viz. " That one Dr. Craig, a Scotchman, coming out of Denmark into his own country, called upon Joh. Neper baron of Marcheston near Edenburg, and told him, among other discourses, of a new invention in Denmark (by Longomontanus as 'tis said) to save the tedious multiplication and division in astronomical calculations. Neper being solicitous to know farther of him concerning this matter, he could give no other account of it, than that it was by proportional numbers. Which hint Neper taking, he desired him at his return to call upon him again. Craig, after some weeks had passed, did so, and Neper then showed him a rude draught of that he called *Canon mirabilis Logarithmorum*. Which draught, with some alterations, he printing in 1614, it came forthwith into the hands of our author Briggs, and into those of Will. Oughtred, from whom the relation of this matter came."

Kepler also says, that one Juste Byrge, assistant astronomer to the landgrave of Hesse, invented or projected logarithms long before Neper did; but that they had never come abroad, on account of the great reservedness of their author with regard to his own compositions. It is also said that Byrge computed a table of natural sines for every two seconds of the quadrant.

But whatever may have been said, or conjectured, concerning any thing that may have been done by others, it is certain that the world is indebted, for the first publication of logarithms, to John Napier, or Nepair*, or in Latin, Neper, baron of Merchiston, or Markinston,

---

* The origin of which name, Crawfurd informs us, was from a (less) peer*less* action of one of his ancestors, viz. Donald, second son of the earl of Lenox, in the time of David the Second. " Some English writers, mistaking the import of the term *baron*, have called this celebrated person lord Napier, a Scotch nobleman. He was not indeed a peer of Scotland: but the peerage of Scotland informs us, that he was of a very ancient, honourable, and illustrious family; that his ancestors, for many generations, had been possessed of sundry baronies, and, amongst others, of the barony of Merchistoun, which descended to him by the death of his father in 1608. Mr. Briggs, therefore, very properly styles him *Baro Merchestonii*. Now, according to Skene, *de verborum significatione*, ' In this realm (of Scotland) he is called a Barronne, quha haldis his landes immediatelie in chief of the king, and hes power of Pit and Gallows; *Fossa et Furca*; quhilk was first institute and granted be king Malcome, quha gave power to the Barrones to have ane Pit, quhairin women condemned for thieft suld be drowned, and ane Gallows, whereupon men thieves and trespassowres suld be hanged, conforme to the doome given in the Barron Court thereanent.' So that a Scotch baron, though no peer, was nevertheless a very considerable personage, both in dignity and power." *Read's Essay on Logarithms*... The name of the illustrious inventor of logarithms, and his family, has been variously written at different times, and on different occasions. In his own Latin works, and in (perhaps) all other books in Latin, it is *Neper*, or *Neperus Baro Merchestonii*; By Briggs, in a letter to Archbishop Usher, he is called *Neper lord of Markinston:* In Wright's translation of the Logarithms, which was revised by the author himself, and published in 1616, he is called *Nepair, baron of Marchiston;* and the same by Crawfurd and some others: But M'Kenzie and others write it *Napier, baron of Merchiston;* which being also the orthography now used by the family, I shall adopt in this work. I observe also, that the Scotch Compendium of Honour says he was only

in Scotland, who died the 3d of April 1618, at 67 years of age. Baron Napier added considerable improvements to trigonometry, and the frequent numeral computations he performed in this branch gave occasion to his invention of logarithms, in order to save part of the trouble attending those calculations: and for this reason he adapted his tables peculiarly to trigonometrical uses.

This discovery he published in 1614, in his book intitled *Mirifici Logarithmorum Canonis Descriptio*, reserving the construction of the numbers till the sense of the learned concerning his invention should be known. And, excepting the construction, this is a perfect work on this kind of logarithms, containing in effect the logarithms of all numbers, and the logarithmic sines, tangents, and secants, for every minute of the quadrant, together with the description and uses of the tables, as also his definition and idea of logarithms.

Napier explains his notion of logarithms by lines described or generated by the motion of points, in this manner: He first conceives a line to be generated by the equable motion of a point, which passes over equal portions of it in equal small moments or portions of time: he then considers another line as generated by the unequal motion of a point, in such manner that, in the aforesaid equal moments or portions of time, there may be described or cut off, from a given line, parts which shall be continually in the same proportion with the respective remainders, of that line, which had before been left: then are the several lengths of the first line, the logarithms of the corresponding parts of the latter. Which description of them is similar to this, that the logarithms are a series of quantities or numbers in arithmetical progression, adapted to another series in geometrical progression. The first or whole length of the line, which is diminished in geometrical progression, he makes the radius of a circle, and its logarithm 0 or nothing, representing the beginning of the first or arithmetical line ; and the several proportional remainders of the geometrical line, are the natural sines of all the other parts of the quadrant, decreasing down to nothing, while the successive increasing values of the arithmetical line, are the corresponding logarithms of those decreasing sines: so that, while the natural lines decrease from radius to nothing, their logarithms increase from nothing to infinite. Napier made the logarithm of radius to be 0, that he might save the trouble of adding and subtracting it, in trigonometrical proportions, in which it so frequently occurred; and he made the logarithms of the sines, from the entire quadrant down to 0, to increase, that they might be positive, and so in his opinion the easier to manage, the sines being of more frequent use than the tangents and secants, of which the whole of the latter and half the former would, in his way, be of a different affection from the sines ; for it is evident that the logarithms of all the secants in the quadrant, and of all the tangents above 45°, or the half quadrant, would be negative, being the logarithms of numbers greater than the radius, whose logarithm is made equal to 0 or nothing.

Sir John Napier, and that his son and heir Archibald, was the first lord, being raised to that dignity in 1626. Be this however as it may, I shall conform to the common modes of expression, and call him indifferently, *Baron Napier*, or *Lord Napier*.

E

As to the contents of Napier's table; it consists of the natural sines and their logarithms, for every minute of the quadrant. Like most other tables, the arcs are continued to 45 degrees from top to bottom on the left-hand side of the pages, and then returned backwards from bottom to top on the right-hand side of the pages: so that the arcs and their complements, with the sines, natural and logarithmic, stand on the same line of the page, in six columns; and in another column, in the middle of the page, are placed the differences between the logarithmic sines and cosines on the same lines, and in the adjacent columns on the right and left; thus making in all seven columns in each page. Of these columns, the first and seventh contain the arc and its complement, in degrees and minutes; the second and sixth, the natural sine and cosine of each arc; the third and fifth, the logarithmic sine and cosine; and the fourth, or middle column, the difference between the logarithmic sine and cosine which are in the third and fifth columns. To elucidate the description, the first page of the table is here inserted, as follows:

Gr. min.	0 Sinus.	Logarithmi.	+ | − Differentiæ.	Logarithmi.	Sinus.	
0	0	Infinitum.	Infinitum.	0	10000000	60
1	2909	81425681	81425680	1	10000000	59
2	5818	74494213	74494211	2	9999998	58
3	8727	70439564	70439560	4	9999996	57
4	11636	67562746	67562739	7	9999993	56
5	14544	65331315	65331304	11	9999989	55
6	17453	63508099	63508083	16	9999984	54
7	20362	61966595	61966573	22	9999980	53
8	23271	60631284	60631256	28	9999974	52
9	26180	59453453	59453418	35	9999967	51
10	29088	58399857	58399814	43	9999959	50
11	31997	57446759	57446707	52	9999950	49
12	34906	56576646	56576584	62	9999940	48
13	37815	55776222	55776149	73	9999928	47
14	40724	55035148	55035064	84	9999917	46
15	43632	54345225	54345129	96	9999905	45
16	46541	53699843	53699734	109	9999892	44
17	49450	53093600	53093577	123	9999878	43
18	52359	52522019	52521881	138	9999863	42
19	55268	51981356	51981202	154	9999847	41
20	58177	51468431	51468361	170	9999831	40
21	61086	50980537	50980450	187	9999813	39
22	63995	50515342	50515137	205	9999795	38
23	66904	50070827	50070603	224	9999776	37
24	69813	49645239	49644995	244	9999756	36
25	72721	49237030	49236765	265	9999736	35
26	75630	48844826	48844539	287	9999714	34
27	78539	48467431	48467122	309	9999692	33
28	81448	48103763	48103431	332	9999668	32
29	84357	47752859	47752503	336	9999644	31
30	87265	47413852	47413471	381	9999619	30

Besides the columns which are actually contained in this table, as above exhibited and described, namely, the natural and logarithmic sines and their differences, the same table is made to serve also for the logarithmic tangents and secants of the whole quadrant, and for the logarithms of common numbers. For, the fourth or middle column contains the logarithmic tangents, being equal to the differences between the logarithmic sines and cosines, when the logarithm of radius is 0, because cosine : sine :: radius : tangent, that is, in logarithms, tangent = sine — cosine. Also the logarithmic sines, made negative, become the logarithmic cosecants, and the logarithmic cosines made negative, are the logarithmic secants; because sine : radius :: radius : cosecant, and cosine : radius :: radius : secant; that is, in logarithms, cosecant = 0 — sine = — sine, and secant = 0 — cosine = — cosine. And to make it answer the purpose of a table of logarithms of common numbers, the author directs to proceed thus: A number being given, find that number in any table of natural sines, or tangents, or secants, and note the degrees and minutes in its arc: then in his table find the corresponding logarithmic sine, or tangent, or secant, to the same number of degrees and minutes; and it will be the required logarithm of the given number.

After his definitions and descriptions of logarithms, Napier explains his table, and illustrates the precepts with examples, showing how to take out the logarithms of sines, tangents, secants, and of common numbers; as also how to add and subtract logarithms. He then proceeds to teach the uses of those numbers; and first, in finding any of the terms of three or four proportionals, showing how to multiply and divide, and to find powers and roots, by logarithms: 2dly, in trigonometry, both plane and spherical, but especially the latter, in which he is very explicit, turning all the theorems for every case into logarithms, computing examples to each in numbers, and then enumerating a set of astronomical problems of the sphere which properly belong to each case. Napier here teaches also some new theorems in spherical trigonometry, particularly, that the tangent of half the base : tang. $\frac{1}{2}$ sum legs :: tang. $\frac{1}{2}$ dif. legs : tang. $\frac{1}{2}$ the alternate base; and the general theorem for what are called his five circular parts, by which he condenses into one rule, in two parts, the theorems for all the cases of right-angled spherical triangles, which had been separately demonstrated by Pitiscus, Lansbergius, Copernicus, Regiomontanus, and others.

The description and use of Napier's canon being in the Latin language, they were translated into English by Mr. Edward Wright, an ingenious mathematician, and inventor of the principles of what has commonly, though erroneously, been called Mercator's Sailing. He sent the translation to the author, at Edinburgh, to be revised by him before publication; who having carefully perused it, returned it with his approbation, and a few lines introduced besides into the translation. But, Mr. Wright dying soon after he received it back, it was after his death published, together with the tables, but each

number to one figure less, in the year 1616, by his son, Samuel
Wright, accompanied with a dedication to the East India Company,
as also a preface by Henry Briggs, of whom we shall presently have
occasion to speak more at large, on account of the great share he bore
in perfecting the logarithms.   In this translation, Mr. Briggs gave
also the description and draught of a scale that had been invented by
Mr. Wright, and several other methods of his own, for finding the proportional parts to intermediate numbers, the logarithms having been
only printed for such numbers as were the natural sines of each
minute.   And the note which Baron Napier inserted in this English
edition, and which was not in the original, was as follows : " But be-
" cause the addition and subtraction of these former numbers may seem
" somewhat painfull, I intend (if it shall please God) in a second edition,
" to set out such logarithms as shall make those numbers above written
" to fall upon decimal numbers, such as 100,000,000, 200,000,000
" 300,000,000 &c, which are easie to be added or abated to or from
" any other number."   This note had reference to the alteration of the
scale of logarithms, in such manner, that 1 should become the logarithm of the ratio of 10 to 1, instead of the number 2·3025851, which
Napier had made that logarithm in his table, and which alteration had
before been recommended to him by Briggs, as we shall see presently.
Napier also inserted a similar remark in his *Rabdologia,* which he
printed at Edinburgh in 1617.

   The following is the preface to Wright's * book, which, as far as

---

* Of this ingenious man I shall here insert in a note the following memoirs, as they have
been translated from a Latin piece taken out of the annals of Gonvile and Caius College at
Cambridge, viz. " This year (1615) died at London, Edward Wright of Garveston in Norfolk,
formerly a fellow of this college ; a man respected by all for the integrity and simplicity of his
manners, and also famous for his skill in the mathematical sciences : insomuch that he was
deservedly styled a most excellent mathematician by Richard Hackluyt, the author of an original
treatise of our English navigations.   What knowledge he had acquired in the science of
mechanics, and how usefully he employed that knowledge to the public as well as private advantage, abundantly appear both from the writings he published, and from the many mechanical
operations still extant, which are standing monuments of his great industry and ingenuity.   He
was the first undertaker of that difficult but useful work, by which a little river is brought from
the town of Ware in a new canal, to supply the city of London with water ; but by the tricks of
others he was hindered from completing the work he had begun.   He was excellent both in
contrivance and execution ; nor was he inferior to the most ingenious mechanic in the making of
instruments, either of brass, or any other matter.   To his invention is owing whatever advantage
Hondius's geographical charts have above others ; for it was our Wright that taught Jodocus
Hondius the method of constructing them, which was till then unknown : but the ungrateful
Hondius concealed the name of the true author, and arrogated the glory of the invention to himself.   Of this fraudulent practice the good man could not help complaining, and justly enough,
in the preface to his Treatise of the Correction of Errors in the Art of Navigation ; which he
composed with excellent judgement, and after long experience, to the great advancement of naval
affairs.   For the improvement of this art he was appointed mathematical lecturer by the East-
India Company, and read lectures in the house of that worthy knight Sir Thomas Smith, for
which he had a yearly salary of fifty pounds.   This office he discharged with great reputation,
and much to the satisfaction of his hearers.   He published in English, a book on the doctrine of
the sphere, and another concerning the construction of sun-dials.   He also prefixed an ingenious
preface to the learned Gilbert's book on the load-stone.   By these and other his writings, he has
transmitted his fame to latest posterity.   While he was yet a fellow of this college, he could not
be concealed in his private study, but was called forth to the public business of the kingdom, by

where it mentions the change from the Latin into English, is a literal translation of the preface to Napier's original; but what follows that, is added by Napier himself. And I willingly insert it here, as it contains a declaration of the motives which led to this discovery, and as the book itself is very scarce. " Seeing there is nothing (right well beloved students in the mathematics) that is so troublesome to Mathematicall practise, nor that doth more molest and hinder Calculators, than the Multiplications, Divisions, square and cubical Extractions of great numbers, which, besides the tedious expence of time, are for the most part subject to many slippery errors: I began therefore to consider in my minde, by what certaine and ready Art I might remove those hindrances. And having thought upon many things to this purpose, I found at length some excellent briefe rules to be treated of (perhaps) hereafter. But amongst all, none more profitable than this, which together with the hard and tedious Multiplications, Divisions, and Extractions of rootes, doth also cast away from the worke it selfe, even the very numbers themselves that are to be multiplied, divided, and resolved into rootes, and putteth other numbers in their place, which performe as much as they can do, onely by Addition and Subtraction, Division by two, or Division by three; which secret invention, being (as all other good things are) so much the better as it shall be the more common; I thought good heretofore to set forth in Latine for the publique use of Mathematicians. But now some of our Countrymen in this Island well affected to these studies, and the more publique good, procured a most learned Mathematician to translate the same into our vulgar English tongue, who after he had finished it sent the Coppy of it to me, to be seene and considered on by myself. I having most willingly and gladly done the same, finde it to be most exact and precisely conformable to my minde and the originall. Therefore it may please you who are inclined to these studies, to receive it from me and the Translator, with as much good will as we recommend it unto you. Fare yee well."

There are also extant copies of Wright's translation with the date 1618 in the title: but this is not properly a new edition, being only the old work with a new title-page adapted to it (the old one being cancelled), together with the addition of sixteen pages of new matter, called

---

the queen's majesty, about the year 1593. He was ordered to attend the earl of Cumberland in some maritime expeditions. One of these he has given a faithful account of, in the way of a journal or ephemeris, to which he has prefixed an elegant hydrographical chart of his own contrivance. A little before his death, he employed himself about an English translation of the book of logarithms then lately found out by the honourable Baron Napier, a Scotchman, who had a great affection for him. This posthumous work of his was published soon after, by his only son Samuel Wright, who was also a scholar of this college. He had formed many other useful designs, but was hindered by death from bringing them to perfection. Of him it may be truly said, that he studied more to serve the public than himself; and though he was rich in fame, and in the promises of the great, yet he died poor, to the scandal of an ungrateful age."

Other anecdotes of him, as well as many other mathematical authors, may be found in the curious history of navigation by Dr. James Wilson, prefixed to Mr. Robertson's excellent treatise on that subject.

" An Appendix to the Logarithms, showing the practice of the calcu-lation of triangles, and also a new and ready way for the exact finding out of such lines and logarithms as are not precisely to be found in the canons." But we are not told by what author : probably it was by Briggs.

Besides the trouble attending Napier's canon, in finding the propor-tional parts, when used as a table of the logarithms of common num-bers, and which was in part remedied by the fore-mentioned con-trivances of Wright and Briggs, it was also accompanied with another inconvenience, which arose from the logarithms being sometimes $+$ or additive, and sometimes $-$ or negative, and which required there-fore the knowledge of algebraical addition and subtraction. And this inconvenience was occasioned, partly by making the logarithm of radius to be 0, and the sines to decrease, and partly by the compendious manner in which the author had formed the table; making the three columns of sines, cosines, and tangents, to serve also for the other three of cosecants, secants, and cotangents.

But this latter inconvenience was well remedied by John Speidell, in his *New Logarithms*, first published in 1619, which contained all the six columns, and in this order; sines, cosines, tangents, cotangents, secants, cosecants : and they were besides made all positive, by being taken the arithmetical complements of Napier's, that is, they were the remainders left by subtracting each of these latter from 10000000. And the former inconvenience was more effectually removed by the said Speidell, in an additional table, given in the sixth impression of the former work, in the year 1624. This was a table of Napier's logarithms for the round or integer numbers 1, 2, 3, 4, 5, &c, to 1000, together with the differences and arithmetical complements; as also the halves of the said logarithms, with their differences and arithme-tical complements; which halves consequently were the logarithms of the square roots of the said numbers. These logarithms are however a little varied in their form from Napier's, namely, so as to increase *from* 1, whose logarithm is 0, instead of decreasing *to* 1, or radius, whose logarithm Napier made 0 likewise; that is, Speidell's logarithm of any number n, is equal to Napier's logarithm of its reciprocal $\frac{1}{n}$: so that in this last table of Speidell's, the logarithm of 1 being 0, the logarithm of 10 is 2302584, the logarithm of 100 is twice as much, or 4605168, and that of 1000 thrice as much, or 6907753.

This table is now commonly called *hyperbolic* logarithms, because the numbers express the areas between the asymptote and curve of the hyperbola, those areas being limited by ordinates parallel to the other asymptote, and the ordinates decreasing in geometrical progression. But this is not a very proper method of denominating them, as such areas may be made to denote any system of logarithms whatever, as we shall show more at large in the proper place.

In the year 1619, Robert Napier, son of the inventor of logarithms, published a new edition of his late father's *Logarithmorum Canonis Descriptio*, together with the promised *Logarithmorum Canonis Con-*

structio, and other miscellaneous pieces, written by his father and by Mr. Briggs.—Also one Bartholomew Vincent, a bookseller at Lugdunum, or Lyons, in France, printed there an exact copy of the same two works in one volume, in the year 1620; which was four years before the logarithms were carried to France by Wingate, who was therefore erroneously said to have first introduced them into that country. But I shall treat more particularly of the contents of this work, after having enumerated the other writers on this kind of logarithms.

In 1618 or 1619, Benjamin Ursinus, mathematician to the Elector of Brandenburgh, published, at Cologn, his *Cursus Mathematicus,* in which is contained a copy of Napier's logarithms, with the addition of some tables of proportional parts. And in 1624, he printed at the same place, his *Trigonometria,* with a table of natural sines and their logarithms, of the Napierian kind and form, to every ten seconds in the quadrant; which he had been at much pains in computing.

In the same year 1624, logarithms, of nearly the same kind, were also published, at Marpurg, by the celebrated John Kepler, mathematician to the Emperor Ferdinand the Second, under the title of *Chilias Logarithmorum ad Totidem Numeros Rotundos, præmissa Demonstratione legitima Ortus Logarithmorum eorumque Usus, &c;* and the year following, a supplement to the same; being applied to round or integer numbers, and to such natural sines as nearly coincide with them. These are exactly the same kind of logarithms as Napier's, being the same logarithms of the natural sines of arcs, beginning from the quadrant, whose sine or radius is 10,000,000, the logarithm of which is made 0, and from thence the sines decreasing by equal differences, down to 0, or the beginning of the quadrant, while their logarithms increase to infinity. So that the difference between this table and Napier's, consists only in this, namely, that in Napier's table the *arc* of the quadrant is divided into equal parts, differing by one minute each, and consequently their sines, to which the logarithms are adapted, are irrational or interminate numbers, and only expressed by approximate decimals; whereas in Kepler's table, the *radius* is divided into equal parts, which are considered as perfect and terminate sines, having equal differences, and to which terminate sines the logarithms are here adapted. By this means indeed the proportions for intermediate numbers and logarithms are easier made, but then the corresponding arcs are not terminate, but irrational, and only set down to an approximate degree. So that Kepler's table is more convenient as a table of the logarithms of common numbers, and Napier's as the logarithmic sines of the arcs of the quadrant. In both tables, the logarithm of the ratio of 10 to 1, is the same quantity, namely 23025852; and as the radius, or greatest sine, is 10,000,000, whose logarithm is made 0, the logarithms of the decuple parts of it will be found by adding 23025852 continually, or multiplying this logarithm by 2, 3, 4, &c; and hence the logarithm of 1, the first number, or smallest sine, in the table, is 161180959, or 7 times 2302 &c.

Besides the two columns, of the natural sines and their logarithms, with the differences of the logarithms, this table of Kepler's consists also of three other columns; the first of which contains the nearest arcs, belonging to those sines, expressed in degrees, minutes and seconds; and the other two express what parts of the radius each sine is equal to, namely, the one of them in 24th parts of the radius, and minutes and seconds of them; and the other in 60th parts of the radius, and minutes of them. As a specimen I have here extracted the last page of the table printed exactly as in the work:

Arcus Circuli cum differentiis.			Sinus seu numeri absoluti.	Partes vicesimæ quartæ.			Logarithmi cum differentiis.	Partes sexagenariæ.	
	19.	34					101.58		
80.	3.	46	98500.00	23.	38.	24	1511.36+	59.	6
	20.	12					101.47		
80.	23.	58	98600.00	23.	39.	50	1409.89+	59.	10
	20.	53					101.37		
80.	44.	51	98700.00	23.	41.	17	1308.52+	59.	13
	21.	42					101.26		
81.	6.	33	98800.00	23.	42.	43	1207.26	59.	17
	22.	53					101.17		
81.	29.	26	98900.00	23.	44.	10	1106.09+	59.	20
	24.	6					101.06		
81.	53.	32	99000.00	23.	45.	36	1005.03+	59.	24
	25.	6					100.96		
82.	18.	38	99100.00	23.	47.	2	904.07+	59.	28
	26.	28					100.85		
82.	45.	6	99200.00	23.	48.	29	803.22+	59.	31
	27.	54					100.76		
83.	13.	0	99300.00	23.	49.	55	702.46	59.	35
	30.	20					100.65		
83.	43.	20	99400.00	23.	51.	22	601.81	59.	38
	32.	40					100.56		
84.	16.	0	99500.00	23.	52.	48	501.25+	59.	42
	36.	30					100.45		
84.	52.	30	99600.00	23.	54.	14	400.80	59.	46
	41.	9					100.35		
85.	33.	39	99700.00	23.	55.	41	300.45	59.	49
	48.	54					100.25		
86.	22.	33	99800.00	23.	57.	7	200.20	59.	53
— 1.	3.	42					100.15		
87.	26.	15	99900.00	23.	58.	34	100.05	59.	56
2.	33.	45					100.05		
90.	0.	0.	100000.00	24.	0.	0	000000.00	60.	0

To the table, Kepler prefixes a pretty considerable tract, containing the construction of the logarithms, and a demonstration of their properties and structure, in which he considers logarithms, in the true and legitimate way, as the measures of ratios, as shall be shown more particularly hereafter in the next part, where we shall treat of the construction of logarithms.

Kepler also introduced the logarithmic calculus into his Rudolphine tables, published in 1627; and inserted in that work several logarithmic tables; as, first, a table similar to that above described, except that the second, or column of sines, or of absolute numbers, is omitted, and, instead of it, another column is added, showing what part of the quadrant each arc is equal to, namely the quotient, expressed in integers and sexagesimal parts, arising from the dividing the whole quadrant by each given arc; 2dly, Napier's table of logarithmic sines to every minute of the quadrant; also two other smaller tables, adapted for the purposes of eclipses and the latitudes of the planets. In this work also Kepler gives a succinct account of logarithms, with the description and use of those that are contained in these tables. And here it is that he mentions Justus Byrgius, as having had logarithms before Napier published them.

Besides the above, some few others published logarithms of the same kind about this time. But let us now return to treat of the history of the common or Briggs's logarithms, so called because he first computed them, and first mentioned them, and recommended them to Napier, instead of the first kind by him invented.

Mr. Henry Briggs, not less esteemed for his great probity, and other eminent virtues, than for his excellent skill in mathematics, was at the time of the publication of Napier's logarithms, in 1614, professor of geometry in Gresham college in London, having been appointed the first professor after its institution: which appointment he held till January 1620, when he was chosen, also the first, Savilian professor of Geometry at Oxford, where he died January the 26th, 168$\frac{0}{1}$, aged about 74 years.

On the publication of Napier's logarithms, Briggs immediately applied himself to the study and improvement of them. In a letter to Mr. (afterwards Archbishop) Usher, dated the 10th of March 1615, he writes, " that he was wholly taken up and employed about the noble invention of logarithms, lately discovered." And again, " Napier lord of Markinston hath set my head and hands at work with his new and admirable logarithms: I hope to see him this summer, if it please God; for I never saw a book which pleased me better, and made me more wonder." Thus we find that Briggs began very early to compute logarithms: but these were not of the same kind with Napier's, in which the logarithm of the ratio of 10 to 1 was 2·3025851 &c; for, in Briggs's first attempt he made 1 the logarithm of that ratio; and, from the evidence we have, it appears that he was the first person who formed the idea of this change in the scale, which he presently and liberally communicated, both to the public in his lectures, and to lord Napier himself, who afterwards said that he also had thought of the same thing; as appears by the following extract, translated from

F

the preface to Briggs's *Arithmetica Logarithmica*: " Wonder not (says he) that these logarithms are different from those which the excellent baron of *Marchiston* published in his Admirable Canon. For when I explained the doctrine of them to my auditors at Gresham college in London, I remarked that it would be much more convenient, the logarithm of the sine total or radius being 0 (as in the *Canon Mirificus*), if the logarithm of the-10th part of the said radius, namely, of 5° 44' 21″, were 100000 &c; and concerning this I presently wrote to the author; also, as soon as the season of the year and my public teaching would permit, I went to Edinburgh, where being kindly received by him, I staid a whole month. But when we began to converse about the alteration of them, he said that he had formerly thought of it, and wished it; but that he chose to publish those that were already done, till such time as his leisure and health would permit him to make others more convenient. And as to the nature of the change, he thought it more expedient that 0 should be made the logarithm of 1: and 100000 &c. the logarithm of radius; which I could not but acknowledge was much better. Therefore, rejecting those which I had before prepared, I proceeded, at his exhortation, to calculate these: and the next summer I went again to Edinburgh, to show him the principle of them; and should have been glad to do the same the third summer, if it had pleased God to spare him so long."

So that it is plain that Briggs was the inventor of the present scale of logarithms, in which 1 is the logarithm of the ratio of 10 to 1, and 2 that of 100 to 1, &c; and that the share which Napier had in them, was only advising Briggs to begin at the lowest number 1, and make the logarithms, or artificial numbers, as Napier had also called them, to *increase* with the natural numbers, instead of *decreasing*; which made no alteration in the figures that expressed Briggs's logarithms, but only in their affection or signs, changing them from negative to positive; so that Briggs's first logarithms to the numbers in the second column of the annexed tablet, would have been as in the first column; but after they were changed, as they are here in the third column; which is a change of no essential difference, as the logarithm of the ratio of 10 to 1, the radix of the natural system of numbers, continues the same, a change in the logarithm of that ratio being the only circumstance that can essentially alter the system of logarithms, the logarithm of 1 being 0. And the reason why Briggs, after that interview, rejected what he had before done, and began anew, was probably because he had adapted his new logarithms to the approximate sines of arcs instead of the round or integer numbers, and not from their being logarithms of another system, as were those of Napier.

B	Num.	N
n	10^n	$-n$
3	·001	—3
2	·01	—2
1	·:	—1
0	1	0
—1	10	1
—2	100	2
—3	1000	3
$-n$	10^n	n

On Briggs's return from Edinburgh to London the second time, namely, in 1617, he printed the first thousand logarithms, to eight places of figures, besides the index, under the title of *Logarithmorum Chilias Prima*. But these seem not to have been published till after the death of Napier, which happened on the 3d of April 1618, as before said; for, in the preface to them, Briggs says, " Why these logarithms differ from those set forth by their most illustrious inventor, of ever respectful memory, in his *Canon Mirificus*, IT IS TO BE HOPED his posthumous work will shortly make appear." And as Napier, after communication had with Briggs, on the subject of altering the scale of logarithms, had given notice, both in Wright's translation, and in his own *Rabdologia*, printed in 1617, of his intention to alter the scale (though it appears very plainly that he never intended to compute any more), without making any mention of the share which Briggs had in the alteration, this gentleman modestly gave the above hint. But not finding any regard paid to it in the said posthumous work, published by lord Napier's son in 1619, where the alteration is again adverted to, but still without any mention of Briggs; this gentleman thought he could not do less than state the grounds of that alteration himself, as they are above extracted from his work pub lished in 1624.

Thus, upon the whole matter, it seems evident that Briggs, whether he had thought of this improvement in the construction of logarithms, of making 1 the logarithm of the ratio of 10 to 1, before lord Napier, or not (which is a secret that could be known only to Napier himself), was the first person who communicated the idea of such an improvement to the world; and that he did this in his lectures to his auditors at Gresham college in the year 1615, very soon after his perusal of Napier's *Canon Mirificus Logarithmorum* in the year 1614. He also mentioned it to Napier, both by letter in the same year, and on his first visit to him in Scotland in the summer of the year 1616, when Napier approved the idea, and said it had already occurred to himself, and that he had determined to adopt it. It would therefore have been more candid in lord Napier to have told the world, in the second edition of this book, that Mr. Briggs had mentioned this improvement to him, and that he had thereby been confirmed in the resolution he had already taken, before Mr. Briggs's communication with him (if indeed that was the fact), to adopt it in that his second edition, as being better fitted to the decimal notation of arithmetic which was in general use. Such a declaration would have been but an act of justice to Mr. Briggs; and the not having made it, cannot but incline us to suspect that lord Napier was desirous that the world should ascribe to him alone the merit of this very useful improvement of the logarithms, as well as that of having originally invented them; though, if the having first communicated an invention to the world be sufficient to entitle a man to the honour of having first invented it, Mr. Briggs had the better title to be called the first inventor of this happy improvement of logarithms.

In 1620, two years after the *Chilias Prima* of Briggs came out, Mr. Edmund Gunter published his *Canon of Triangles*, which contains the artificial or logarithmic sines and tangents, for every minute, to seven places of figures, besides the index, the logarithm of radius being 10·0 &c. These logarithms are of the kind last agreed upon by Napier and Briggs, and they were the first tables of logarithmic sines and tangents that were published of this sort. Gunter also, in 1623, reprinted the same in his book *De Sectore et Radio*, together with the *Chilias Prima* of his old colleague Mr. Briggs, he being professor of astronomy at Gresham college when Briggs was professor of geometry there, Gunter having been elected to that office the 6th of March 1619, and enjoyed it till his death, which happened on the 10th of December, 1626, about the forty-fifth year of his age. In 1623 also, Gunter applied these logarithms of numbers, sines, and tangents, to straight lines drawn on a ruler; with which, proportions in common numbers and trigonometry were resolved by the mere application of a pair of compasses; a method founded on this property, that the logarithms of the terms of equal ratios are equidifferent. This instrument, in the form of a two-foot scale, is now in common use for navigation, and other purposes, and is commonly called the Gunter. He also greatly improved the sector for the same uses. Gunter was the first who used the word *co-sine* for the sine of the complement of an arc. He also introduced the use of arithmetical complements into the logarithmical arithmetic, as is witnessed by Briggs, chap. XV. Arith. Log. And it has been said, that he started the idea of the logarithmic curve, which was so called because the segments of its axis are the logarithms of the corresponding ordinates.

The logarithmic lines were afterwards drawn in various other ways. In 1627, they were drawn by Wingate on two separate rulers sliding against each other, to save the use of compasses in resolving proportions. They were also, in 1627, applied to concentric circles, by Oughtred. Then in a spiral form by a Mr. Milburne of Yorkshire about the year 1650. And, lastly, in 1657, on the present sliding rule, by Seth Partridge.

The discoveries relating to logarithms were carried to France by Mr. Edmund Wingate, but not first of all, as he erroneously says in the preface to his book. He published at Paris, in 1624, two small tracts in the French language: and afterwards at London, in 1626, an English edition of the same, with improvements. In the first of these, he teaches the use of Gunter's ruler; and in the other, that of Briggs's logarithms, and the artificial sines and tangents. Here are contained also, tables of those logarithms, sines, and tangents, copied from Gunter. The edition of these logarithms printed at London in 1635, and the former editions also, I suppose, has the units figures disposed along the tops of the columns, and the tens down the margins, like our tables at present; with the whole logarithm, which was only to six places of figures, in the angle of meeting: which is the first instance that I have seen of this mode of arrangement.

But proceed we now to the larger structure of logarithms.

Briggs had continued from the beginning to labour with great industry at the computation of those logarithms of which he before published a short specimen in small numbers. And, in 1624, he produced his *Arithmetica Logarithmica*—a stupendous work for so short a time!—containing the logarithms of 30000 natural numbers, to fourteen places of figures besides the index, namely, from 1 to 20000, and from 90000 to 100000; together with the differences of the logarithms. Some writers say that there was another *chiliad*, namely, from 100000 to 101000; but none of the copies that I have seen have more than the 30000 above mentioned, and they were all regularly terminated in the usual way with the word FINIS. The preface to these logarithms contains, among other things, an account of the alteration made in the scale by Napier and himself, from which we before gave an extract; and an earnest solicitation to others to undertake the computation for the intermediate numbers, offering to give instructions, and paper ready ruled for that purpose, to any persons so inclined to contribute to the completion of so valuable a work. In the introduction, he gives also an ample treatise on the construction and uses of these logarithms, which will be particularly described hereafter.——By this invitation, and other means, he had hopes of collecting materials for the logarithms of the intermediate 70000 numbers, whilst he should employ his own labour more immediately on the canon of logarithmic sines and tangents, and so carry on both works at once; as indeed they were both equally necessary, and he himself was now pretty far advanced in years.

Soon after this, Adrian Vlacq, or Flack, of Gouda in Holland, completed the intermediate seventy chiliads, and republished the *Arithmetica Logarithmica* at that place, in 1627 and 1628, with those intermediate numbers, making in the whole the logarithms of all numbers to 100000, but only to ten places of figures. To these was added a table of artificial sines, tangents, and secants, to every minute of the quadrant.

Briggs himself lived also to complete a table of logarithmic sines and tangents for the hundredth part of every degree, to fourteen places of figures besides the index; together with a table of natural sines for the same parts to fifteen places, and the tangents and secants for the same to ten places; with the construction of the whole. These tables were printed at *Gouda*, under the care of Adrian Vlacq, and mostly finished off before 1631, though not published till 1633. But his death, which then happened, prevented him from completing the application and uses of them. However, the performing of this office, when dying, he recommended to his friend Henry Gellibrand, who was then professor of astronomy in Gresham college, having succeeded Mr. Gunter in that appointment. Gellibrand accordingly added a preface, and the application of the logarithms to plane and spherical trigonometry, &c; and the whole was printed at Gouda by the same printer, and brought out in the same year, 1633, as the *Trigonometria Artificialis* of Vlacq, who had the care of the press as above said. This work was called *Trigonometria Britannica;* and besides the arcs in degrees and centesms of degrees, it has another column, containing the minutes and seconds answering to the several centesms in the first column.

In 1633, as mentioned above, Vlacq printed at Gouda, in Holland, his *Trigonometria Artificialis; sive Magnus Canon Triangulorum Logarithmicus ad Decadas Secundorum Scrupulorum constructus.* This work contains the logarithmic sines and tangents to ten places of figures, with their differences, for every ten seconds in the quadrant. To them is also added Briggs's table of the first 20000 logarithms, but carried only to ten places of figures besides the index, with their differences. The whole is preceded by a description of the tables, and the application of them to plane and spherical trigonometry, chiefly extracted from Briggs's *Trigonometria Britannica*, above mentioned.

Gellibrand published also, in 1635, *An Institution Trigonometricall*, containing the logarithms of the first 10000 numbers, with the natural sines, tangents, and secants, and the logarithmic sines and tangents, for degrees and minutes, all to seven places of figures, besides the index; as also other tables proper for navigation; with the uses of the whole. Gellibrand died the 9th of February 1636, in the 40th year of his age, to the great loss of the mathematical world.

Besides the persons hitherto mentioned, who were mostly computers of logarithms, many others have also published tables of those artificial numbers, more or less complete, and sometimes improved and varied in the manner and form of them. We may here just advert to a few of the principal of these.

In 1626, D. Henrion published, at Paris, a treatise concerning Briggs's logarithms of common numbers from 1 to 20000, to eleven places of figures; with the sines and tangents to eight places only.

In 1631, was printed, at London, by one George Miller, a book containing Briggs's logarithms, with their differences, to ten places of figures besides the index, for all numbers to 100000; as also the logarithmic sines, tangents, and secants, for every minute of the quadrant; with the explanation and uses in English.

The same year, 1631, Richard Norwood published his *Trigonometrie;* in which we find Briggs's logarithms for all numbers to 10000, and for the sines, tangents, and secants, to every minute, both to seven places besides the index.—In the conclusion of the trigonometry, he complains of the unfair practices of printing Vlacq's book in 1627 or 1628, and the book mentioned in the last article. His words are, " Now whereas I have here, and in sundry places in this book, cited Mr. Briggs his *Arithmetica Logarithmica* (lest I may seem to abuse the reader), you are to understand not the book put forth about a month since in English, as a translation of his, and with the same title; being nothing like his, nor worthy his name; but the book which himself put forth with this title in Latin, being printed at London anno 1624. And here I have just occasion to blame the ill dealing of these men, both in the matter before mentioned, and in printing a second edition of his *Arithmetica Logarithmica* in Latin, whilst he lived, against his mind and liking; and brought them over to sell, when the first were unsold; so frustrating those additions which Mr. Briggs intended in his second edition, and moreover leaving out some things that were in the first edition, of special moment: a practice of very ill consequence, and tending to the great disparagement of such as take pains in this kind."

Francis Bonaventure Cavalerius published at Bologna, in 1632, his *Directorium Generale Uranometricum*, in which are tables of Briggs's logarithms of sines, tangents, secants, and versed sines, each to eight places, for every second of the first five minutes, for every five seconds from five to ten minutes, for every ten seconds from ten to twenty minutes, for every twenty seconds from twenty to thirty minutes, for every thirty seconds from 30' to 1° 30', and for every minute in the rest of the quadrant: which is the first table of logarithmic versed sines that I know of. In this book are contained also the logarithms of the first ten chiliads of natural numbers, namely, from 1 to 10000, disposed in this manner: all the twenties at top, and from 1 to 19 on the side, the logarithm of the sum being in the square of meeting. In this work, also, I think Cavalerius gave the method of finding the area or spherical surface contained by various arcs described on the surface of a sphere; which had before been given by Albert Girard, in his Algebra, printed in the year 1629.

Also, in the *Trigonometria* of the same author, Cavalerius, printed in 1643, besides the logarithms of numbers from 1 to 1000, to eight places, with their differences, we find both natural and logarithmic sines, tangents, and secants, the former to seven, and the latter to eight places; namely, to every 10″ of the first 30 minutes, to every 30″ from 30' to 1°; and the same for their complements, or backwards through the last degree of the quadrant; the intermediate 88° being to every minute only.

Mr. Nathaniel Roe, "Pastor of Benacre in Suffolke," also reduced the logarithmic tables to a contracted form, in his *Tabulæ Logarithmicæ*, printed at London in 1633. Here we have Briggs's logarithms of numbers from 1 to 100000, to eight places; the fifties placed at top, and from 1 to 50 on the side; also the first four figures of the logarithms at top, and the other four down the columns. They contain also the logarithmic sines and tangents to every 100th part of degrees, to ten places.

Ludovicus Frobenius published at Hamburg, in 1634, his *Clavis Universa Trigonometriæ*, containing tables of Briggs's logarithms of numbers, from 1 to 2000; and of sines, tangents, and secants, for every minute; both to seven places.

But the table of logarithms of common numbers was reduced to its most convenient form by John Newton, in his *Trigonometria Britannica*, printed at London in 1658, having availed himself of both the improvements of Wingate and Roe, namely, uniting Wingate's disposition of the natural numbers with Roe's contracted arrangement of the logarithms, the numbers being all disposed as in our best tables at present, namely, the units along the top of the page, and the tens down the left-hand side, also the first three figures of each logarithm in the first column, and the remaining five figures in the other columns, the logarithms being to eight places. This work contains also the logarithmic sines and tangents, to eight figures besides the index, for every 100th part of a degree, with their differences, and for 1000th parts in the first three degrees.—In the preface to this work, Newton takes occasion, as Wingate and Norwood had done before, as well as Briggs himself, to censure the unfair practices of some other publishers of logarithms. He says, " In the second part of this institution, thou art presented with Mr. Gellibrand's Trigonometrie, faithfully translated from the Latin copy, that which the author himself published under the title of *Trigonometria Britannica,* and not that which Vlacq the Dutchman styles *Trigonometria Artificialis,* from whose corrupt and imperfect copy that seems to be translated which is amongst us generally known by the name of *Gellibrand's Trigonometry*; but those who either knew him, or have perused his writings, can testify that he was no admirer of the old sexagenary way of working; nay that he did preferre the decimal way before it, as he hath abundantly testified in all the examples of this his trigonometry, which differs from that other which Vlacq hath published, and that which hath hitherto borne his name in English, as in the form, so likewise in the matter of it; for in the two last mentioned editions, there is something left out in the second chapter of plain triangles, the third chapter wholly omitted, and a part of the third in the spherical; but in this edition nothing: something we have added to both, by way of explanation and demonstration."

In 1670, John Caramuel published his *Mathesis Nova*, in which are contained 1000 logarithms both of Napier's and Briggs's form, as also 1000 of what he calls the Perfect Logarithms, namely, the same as those which Briggs first thought of, which differ from the last only in this, that the one increases while the other decreases, the radix or logarithm of the ratio of 10 to 1 being the same in both.

The books of logarithms have since become very numerous, but the logarithms are mostly of that kind invented by Briggs, and which are now in common use. Of these, the most noted for their accuracy or usefulness, besides the works above mentioned, are Vlacq's small volume of tables, particularly that edition printed at Lyons in 1670; also tables printed at the same place in 1760; but most especially the tables of Sherwin and Gardiner. Of these, Sherwin's *Mathematical Tables*, in 8vo. formed the most complete collection of any, containing, besides the logarithms of all numbers to 101000, the sines, tangents, secants, and versed sines, both natural and logarithmic, to every minute of the quadrant. The first edition was in 1706: but the third edition, in 1742, which was revised by Gardiner, is esteemed the most correct of any, though containing many thousands of errors in the final figures: as to the last or fifth edition, in 1771, it is so erroneously printed that no dependance can be placed in it, being the most inaccurate book of tables I ever knew; I have a list of several thousand errors which I have corrected in it, as well as in Gardiner's octavo edition.

Gardiner also printed at London, in 1742, a quarto volume of " Tables of Logarithms, for all numbers from 1 to 102100, and for the sines and tangents to every ten seconds of each degree in the quadrant; as also, for the sines of the first 72 minutes to every single second: with other useful and necessary tables;" namely, a table of Logistical Logarithms, and three smaller tables to be used for finding the logarithms of numbers to twenty places of figures. Of these tables of Gardiner, only a small number was printed, and that by subscription; and they have always been held in great estimation for their accuracy and usefulness.

An edition of Gardiner's collection was also elegantly printed at Avignon in France, in 1770, with some additions, namely, the sines and tangents for every single second in the first four degrees, and a small table of hyperbolic logarithms, copied from a treatise on Fluxions by the late ingenious Mr. Thomas Simpson: but this is not quite so correct as Gardiner's own edition. The tables in all these books are to seven places of figures.

There have also lately appeared the following accurate and elegant books of logarithms; viz.

1. Logarithmic Tables, by the late Mr. Michael Taylor, a pupil of mine, and author of The Sexagesimal Table. His work consists of three tables; 1st. the Logarithms of Common Numbers from 1 to 1260, each to 8 places of figures; 2dly, The Logarithms of all Numbers from 1 to 101000, each to 7 places; 3dly. The Logarithmic Sines and Tangents to every Second of the Quadrant, also to 7 places of figures; a work that must prove highly useful to such persons as may be employed in very nice and accurate calculations, such as astronomical tables, &c. The author dying when the tables were nearly all printed off, the Rev. Dr. Maskelyne, Astronomer Royal, has supplied a preface, containing an account of the work, with excellent precepts for the explanation and use of the tables: the whole very accurately and elegantly printed on large 4to. 1792.

2. " Tables Portatives de Logarithmes, publiées à Londres, par Gardiner," &c. This work is most beautifully printed in a neat portable 8vo volume, and contains all the tables in Gardiner's 4to volume, with some additions and improvements, and with a considerable degree of accuracy. On this, as well as several other occasions, it is but justice to remark the extraordinary spirit and elegance with which the learned men, and the artisans of the French nation, undertake and execute works of merit. Printed at Paris, by Didot, 1793.

3. A second edition of the " Tables Portatives de Logarithmes," &c. printed at Paris with the Stereotypes, of solid pages, in 8vo, 1795, by Didot. This edition is greatly enlarged, by an extension of the old tables and many new ones; among which are the log. sines and tangents to every ten thousandth part of the quadrant, viz. in which the quadrant is first divided into 100 equal parts, and each of these into 100 parts again.

4. Other more extensive tables, not yet quite completed, ordered by the Board of Longitude in France, and under the direction of M. Prony, in which the quadrant is decimally divided into 10000 equal parts.

" The logarithmic canon serves to find readily the logarithm of any assigned number; and we are told by Dr. Wallis, in the second volume of his Mathematical Works, that an antilogarithmic canon, or one to find as readily the number corresponding to every logarithm, was begun, he thinks, by Harriot the algebraist (who died in 1621), and completed by Walter Warner, the editor of Harriot's works, before 1640; which ingenious performance, it seems, was lost, for want of encouragement to publish it."

" A small specimen of such numbers was published in the Philosophical Transactions for the year 1714, by Mr. Long of Oxford; but it was not till 1742 that a complete antilogarithmic canon was published by Mr. James Dodson, wherein he has computed the numbers corresponding to every logarithm from 1 to 100000, for 11 places of figures."

G

THE CONSTRUCTION OF LOGARITHMS, &c.

HAVING described the several kinds of logarithms, their rise and invention, their nature and properties, and given some account of the principal early cultivators of them, with the chief collections that have been published of such tables; proceed we now to deliver a more particular account of the ideas and methods employed by each author, and the peculiar modes of construction made use of by them.

And first, of the great inventor himself, Lord Napier.

Napier's *Construction of Logarithms.*

The Inventor of logarithms did not adapt them to the series of natural numbers 1, 2, 3, 4, 5, &c, as it was not his principal idea to extend them to all arithmetical operations in general; but he confined his labours to that circumstance which first suggested the necessity of the invention, and adapted his logarithms to the approximate numbers which express the natural sines of every minute in the quadrant, as they had been set down by former writers on trigonometry.

The same restricted idea was pursued through his method of constructing the logarithms. As the lines of the sines of all arcs are parts of the radius, or sine of the quadrant, which was therefore called the *sinus totus*, or whole sine, he conceived the line of the radius to be described or run over, by a point moving along it in such a manner, that in equal portions of time it generated, or cut off, parts, in a decreasing geometrical progression, leaving the several remainders, or sines in geometrical progression also; while another point, in an indefinite line, described equal parts of *it* in the same equal portions of time; so that the respective sums of these, or the whole line generated, were always the arithmeticals or logarithms of these sines.

Thus, az is the given radius, on which all the sines are to be taken, and A&c, the indefinite line containing the logarithms; these lines being each generated by the motion of points, beginning at A, a. Now, at the end of the 1st, 2d, 3d, &c, moments, or equal small portions of time, the moving points being found at the places marked 1, 2, 3, &c, then za, z1, z2, z3, &c, will be the series of natural sines, and A 0 (or 0), A1, A2, A3, &c, will be their logarithms; supposing the point which generates az to move every where with a velocity decreasing in proportion to its distance from z, namely, its velocity in the points 0, 1, 2, 3, &c, to be respectively as the distances z0, z1, z2, z3, &c, while the velocity of the point generating the logarithmic line A&c, remains constantly the same as at first in the point A or 0.

Sines.	Log.
a 0	A 0
1	1
2	2
3	3
4	4
5	5
6	6
7	
&c	
	7
z	
	&c

Hitherto the author had not fully limited his system or scale of logarithms, having only supposed one condition or limitation, namely, that the logarithm of the radius az should be 0. Whereas two independent conditions, no matter what, are necessary to limit the scale or system of logarithms. It did not occur to him that it was proper to form the other limit, by affixing some particular value to an assigned number, or part of the radius: but, as another condition was necessary, he assumed *this* for it, namely, that the two generating points should begin to move at a and A with equal velocities; or that the increments a1 and A1, described in the first moments, should be equal; as he thought this circumstance would be attended with some little ease in the computation. And this is the reason that, in his table, the natural sines and their logarithms, at the complete quadrant, have equal differences; and this is also the reason why his scale of logarithms happens accidentally to agree with what have since been called the hyperbolic logarithms, which have numeral differences equal to those of their natural numbers at the beginning; except only that these latter increase with the natural numbers, and his on the contrary decrease; the logarithm of the ratio of 10 to 1 being the same in both, namely 2·30258509.

And here, by the way, it may be observed, that Napier's manner of conceiving the generation of the lines of the natural numbers, and their logarithms, by the motion of points, is very similar to the manner in which Newton afterwards considered the generation of magnitudes in his doctrine of fluxions; and it is also remarkable, that, in art. 2 of the *Habitudines Logarithmorum et suorum naturalium numerorum invicem*, in the appendix to the *Constructio Logarithmorum*, Napier speaks of the velocities of the increments or decrements of the logarithms, in the same way as Newton does of his fluxions, namely, where he shows that those velocities, or fluxions, are inversely as the sines or natural numbers of the logarithms; which is a necessary consequence of the nature of the generation of those lines as described above; with this alteration however, that now the radius az must be considered as generated by an equable motion of the point, and the indefinite line A &c by a motion increasing in the same ratio as the other before decreased; which is a supposition that Napier must have had in view when he stated that relation of the fluxions.

Having thus limited his system, Napier proceeds, in the posthumous work of 1619, to explain his construction of the logarithmic canon; and this he effects in various ways, but chiefly by generating, in a very easy manner, a series of proportional numbers, and their arithmeticals or logarithms; and then finding, by proportion, the logarithms to the natural sines, from those of the nearest numbers among the original proportionals.

After describing the necessary cautions he made use of, to preserve a sufficient degree of accuracy, in so long and complex a process of calculation; such as annexing several ciphers, as decimals separated by a point, to his primitive numbers, and rejecting the decimals thence resulting after the operations were completed; setting the numbers down to the nearest unit in the last figure; and teaching the arithmetical processes of adding, subtracting, multiplying, and dividing the limits between which certain unknown numbers must lie, so as to obtain the limits between which the results must also fall: I say, after describing such particulars, in order to clear and smooth the way, he enters on the great field of calculation itself. Beginning at radius 10000000, he first constructs several descending geometrical series, but of such a nature, that they are all quickly formed by an easy continual subtraction, and a division by 2, or by 10, or 100, &c, which is done by only removing the decimal point so many places towards the left hand, as there are ciphers in the divisor. He constructs three tables of such series: The first of these consist of 100 numbers, in the proportion of radius to radius minus 1, or of 10000000 to 9999999; all of which are found by only subtracting from each its 10000000th part, which part is also found by only removing each figure seven places lower: the last of these 100 proportionals is found to be 9999900·0004950.

The 2d table contains 50 numbers, which are in the continual proportion of the first to the last in the first table, namely, of 10000000·0000000, to 9999900·0004950, or nearly the proportion of 100000 to 99999; these therefore are found by

No.	First Table.	Second Table.
1	10000000.0000000	10000000.000000
2	9999999.0000000	9999900.000000
3	9999998.0000001	9999800.001000
4	9999997.0000003	9999700.003000
&c.	&c till the 100th term, which will be	&c to the 50th term
50		9995001.222927
100	9999900.0004950	

only removing the figures of each number 5 places lower, and subtracting them from the same number: the last of these he finds to be 9995001·222927. And a specimen of these two tables is here annexed.

The 3d table consists of 69 columns, and each column of twenty-one numbers or terms, which, in every column, are in the continual proportion of 10000 to 9995, that is, nearly as the first is to the last in the 2d table; and as 10000 exceeds 9995, by the 2000th part, the terms in every column will be constructed by dividing each upper number by 2, removing the figures of the quotient 3 places lower, and then subtracting them; and in this way it is proper to construct only the first column of 21 numbers, the last of which will be 9900473·5780: but the 1st, 2d, 3d, &c, numbers, in all the columns, are in the continual proportion of 100 to 99, or nearly the proportion of the first to the last in the first column; and therefore these will be found by removing the figures of each preceding number two places lower, and subtracting them, for the like number in the next column. A specimen of this 3d table is as here below.

		THE THIRD TABLE.			
Terms	1st Column.	2d Column.	3d Column.	&c till the	69th Column.
1	10000000.0000	9900000.0000	9801000.0000	&c to	5048858.8900
2	9995000.0000	9895050.0000	9796099.5000	the 4th,	5046334.4605
3	9990002.5000	9890102.4750	9791201.4503	5th, 6th,	5043811.2932
4	9985007.4987	9885157.4237	9786305.8495	7th, &c	5041289.3879
5	9980014.9950	9880214.8451	9781412.6967	col. till	5038768.7435
&c	&c till	&c	&c	the last	&c
21	9900473.5780	9801468.8423	9703454.1539	or	4998609.4034

Thus he had, in this 3d table, interposed between the radius and its half, 68 numbers in the continual proportion of 100 to 99; and interposed between every two of these, 20 numbers in the proportion of 10000 to 9995 : and again, in the 2d table, between 10000000 and 9995000, the two first of the third table, he had 50 numbers in the proportion of 100000 to 99999 ; and lastly, in the 1st table, between 10000000 and 9999900, or the two first in the 2d table, 100 numbers in the proportion of 10000000 to 9999999 ; that is, in all, about 1600 proportionals ; all found in the most simple manner, by little more than easy subtractions ; which proportionals nearly coincide with all the natural sines from 90° down to 30°.

To obtain the logarithms of all those proportionals, he demonstrates several properties and relations of the numbers and logarithms, and illustrates the manner of applying them. The principal of these properties are as follow : 1st, that the logarithm of any sine is greater than the difference between that sine and the radius, but less than the said difference when increased in the proportion of the sine to radius*; and 2dly, that the difference between the logarithms of two sines is less than the difference of the sines increased in the proportion of the less sine to radius, but greater than the said difference of the sines increased in the proportion of the greater sine to radius. †

Hence, by the first theorem, the logarithm of 10000000, the radius or first term in the first table, being 0, the logarithm of 9999999, the 2d term, will be between 1 and 1.0000001, and will therefore be equal to 1.00000005 very nearly : and this will be also the common difference of all the terms or proportionals in the first table : therefore by the continual addition of this logarithm, there will be obtained the logarithms of all these 100 proportionals ; consequently 100 times the said first logarithm, or the last of the above sums, will give 100·000005, for the logarithm of 9999900·0004950, the last of the said 100 proportionals.

Then, by the 2d theorem, it easily appears, that ·0004950 is the difference between the logarithms of 9999900·0004950 and 9999900, the last term of the first table, and the 2d term of the second table ;

---

* By this first theorem, r being radius, the logarithm of the sine s is between $r-s$ and $\dfrac{r-s}{s}r$; and therefore, when s differs but little from r, the logarithm of s will be nearly equal to $\dfrac{(r+s)\times(r-s)}{2s}$, the arithmetical mean between the limits $r-s$ and $\dfrac{r-s}{s}r$; but still nearer to $(r-s)\sqrt{\dfrac{r}{s}}$ or $\dfrac{r-s}{s}\sqrt{rs}$, the geometrical mean between the said limits.

† By this second theorem, the difference between the logarithms of the two sines S and s, lying between the limits $\dfrac{S-s}{s}r$ and $\dfrac{S-s}{S}r$, will, when those sines differ but little, be nearly equal to $\dfrac{S^2-s^2}{2Ss}r$ or $\dfrac{(S+s)\times(S-s)}{2Ss}r$, their arithmetical mean ; or nearly $=\dfrac{S-s}{\sqrt{Ss}}r$, the geometrical mean ; or nearly $=\dfrac{S-s}{S+s}2r$, by substituting in the last denominator, $\frac{1}{2}(S+s)$ for $\sqrt{Ss}$, to which it is nearly equal.

this then being added to the last logarithm, gives 100·0005000 for the logarithm of the said 2d term, as also the common difference of the logarithms of all the proportions in the 2d table; and therefore, by continually adding it, there will be generated the logarithms of all these proportionals in the second table; the last of which is 5000·025, answering to 9995001·222927, the last term of that table.

Again, by the 2d theorem, the difference between the logarithms of this last proportional of the second table, and the 2d term in the first column of the third table, is found to be 1.2235387; which being added to the last logarithm, gives 5001·2485387 for the logarithm of 9995000, the said 2d term of the third table, as also the common difference of the logarithms of all the proportionals in the first column of that table; and that this therefore being continually added, gives all the logarithms of that first column, the last of which is 100024·97077, the logarithm of 9900473.5780, the last term of the said column.

Finally, by the 2d theorem again, the difference between the logarithms of this last number and 9900000, the 1st term in the second column, is 478·3502; which being added to the last logarithm, gives 100503·3210 for the logarithm of the said 1st term in the second column, as well as the common difference of the logarithms of all the numbers on the same line in every line of the table, namely, of all the 1st terms, of all the 2d, of all the 3d, of all the 4th, &c terms in all the columns; and which therefore, being continually added to the logarithms in the first column, will give the corresponding logarithms in all the other columns.

And thus is completed what the author calls the radical table, in which he retains only one decimal place in the logarithms (or *artificials*, as he always call them in his tract on the construction), and four in the naturals. A specimen of the table is as here follows:

RADICAL TABLE.					
Terms	1st Column.		2d Column.		69th Column.
	Naturals.	Artificials	Naturals.	Artificials	Naturals.	Artificials.
1	10000000.0000	0	9900000.0000	100503.3	5048858.8900	6834225.9
2	9995000.0000	5001.2	9895050.0000	105504.6	5046333.4605	6839227.1
3	9990002.5000	10002.5	9890102.4750	110505.8	5043811.2932	6844228.3
4	9985007.4987	15003.7	9885157.4237	115507.1	5041289.3879	6849229.6
5	9980014.9950	20005.0	9880214.8451	120508.3	5038768.7435	6854230.8
&c	&c till	&c	&c	&c	&c	&c
21	9900473.5780	100025.0	9801468.8423	200528.2	4998609.4034	6934250.8

Having thus, in the most easy manner, completed the radical table, by little more than mere addition and subtraction, both for the natural numbers and logarithms; the logarithmic sines were easily deduced from it by means of the 2d theorem, namely, taking the sum and difference of each tabular sine and the nearest number in the radical table, annexing 7 ciphers to the difference, dividing the result by the sum, then half the quotient gives the difference between the logarithms of the said numbers, namely, between the tabular sine and radical number; consequently adding or subtracting this difference, to or from the given logarithm of the radical number, there is obtained the logarithmic sine required. And thus the logarithms 'of all the sines, from radius to the half of it, or from 90° to 30°, were perfected.

Next, for determining the sines of the remaining 30 degrees, he delivers two methods. In the first of these he proceeds in this manner: Observing that the logarithm of the ratio of 2 to 1, or of half the radius, is 6931469·22, of 4 to 1 is the double of this, of 8 to 1 is triple of it, &c; that of 10 to 1 is 23025842·34, of 20 to 1 is the sum of the logarithms of 2 and 10; and so on, by composition for the logarithms of the ratios between 1 and 40, 80, 100, 200, &c; to 10000000; he multiplies any given sine, for an arc less than 30 degrees, by some of these numbers, till he finds the product nearly equal to one of the tabular numbers; then by means of ' this and the second theorem, the logarithm of this product is found; to which adding the logarithm that answers to the multiple above mentioned, the sum is the logarithm sought. But the other method is still much easier, and is derived from this property, which he demonstrates, namely, as half radius is to the sine of half an arc, so is the cosine of the said half arc, to the sine of the whole arc; or as ½ radius : sine of an arc : : cosine of the arc : sine of double arc; hence the logarithmic sine of an arc is found, by adding together the logarithms of half radius and of the sine of the double arc, and then subtracting the logarithmic cosine from the sum.

And thus the remainder of the sines, from 30° down to 0, are easily obtained. But in this latter way, the logarithmic sines for full one half of the quadrant, or from 0 to 45 degrees, he observes, may be derived; the other half having already been made by the general method of the radical table, by one easy division and addition or subtraction for each.

We have dwelt the longer on this work of the inventor of logarithms, because I have not seen, in any author, an account of his method of constructing his table, though it is perfectly different from any other method used by the later computers, and indeed, almost peculiar to his species of logarithms. The whole of this work manifests great ingenuity in the designer, as well as much accuracy. But notwithstanding the caution he took to obtain his logarithms true to the nearest unit in the last figure set down in the tables, by extending the numbers in the computations to several decimals, and other means, he had been disappointed of that end, either by the inaccuracy of his assistant computers or transcribers, or through some other cause; as the logarithms in the table are commonly very inaccurate. It is remarkable too, that in this tract on the construction of the logarithms, Lord Napier never calls them logarithms, but every where *artificials*, as opposed in idea to the natural numbers: and this notion of natural and artificial numbers, I take to have been his first idea of this matter, and that he altered the word *artificials* to *logarithms* in his first book, on the description of them, when he printed it, in the year 1614, and that he would also

have altered the word every where in this posthumous work if he had
lived to print it : for in the two or three pages of appendix, annexed
to the work by his son, from Napier's papers, he again always calls
them logarithms. This appendix relates to the change of the logarithms to that scale in which 1 is the logarithm of the ratio of 10 to 1,
the logarithm of 1, with or without ciphers, being 0; and it appears
to have been written after Briggs communicated to him his idea of
that change.

Napier here in this appendix also briefly describes some methods
by which this new species of logarithms may be constructed. Having
supposed 0 to be the logarithm of 1, and 1, with any number of ciphers,
as 10000000000, the logarithm of 10, he directs to divide this logarithm of 10, and the successive quotients, ten times by 5; by which
divisions there will be obtained these other ten logarithms, namely,
2000000000, 400000000, 80000000, 16000000, 3200000, 640000,
128000, 25600, 5120, 1024 : then this last logarithm, and its quotients, being divided ten times by 2, will give these other ten logarithm, 512, 256, 128, 64, 32, 16, 8, 4, 2, 1. And the numbers
answering to these twenty logarithms we are directed to find in this
manner; namely, extract the 5th root of 10 (with ciphers), then the
5th root of that root, and so on, for ten continual extractions of the
5th root; so shall these ten roots be the natural numbers belonging to
the first ten logarithms, above found in continually dividing by 5 : next,
out of the last 5th root we are to extract the square root, then the
square root of this last root, and so on, for 10 successive extractions
of the square root; so shall these last 10 roots be the natural numbers corresponding to the logarithms or quotients arising from the last
ten divisions by the number 2. And from these twenty logarithms,
1, 2, 4, 8, 16, &c, and their natural numbers, the author observes
that other logarithms and their numbers may be formed, namely, by
adding the logarithms, and multiplying their corresponding numbers.

It is evident that this process would generate rather an antilogarithmic canon, such as Dodson's, than the table of Briggs; and that
the method would also be very laborious, since, besides the very
troublesome original extractions of the 5th roots, all the numbers
would be very large, by the multiplication of which the successive
secondary natural numbers are to be found.

Our author next mentions another method of deriving a few of the
primitive numbers and their logarithms, namely, by taking continually
geometrical means, first between 10 and 1, then between 10 and
this mean, and again between 10 and the last mean, and so on; and
taking the arithmetical means between their corresponding logarithms.
He then lays down various relations between numbers and their logarithms; such as, that the products and quotients of numbers answer
to the sums and differences of their logarithms, and that the powers
and roots of numbers answer to the products and quotients of the
logarithms by the index of the power or root, &c; as also that, of
any two numbers whose logarithms are given, if each number be raised
to the power denoted by the logarithm of the other, the two results

will be equal. He then delivers another method of making the logarithms to a few of the prime integer numbers, which is well adapted for constructing the common table of logarithms. This method easily follows from what has been said above; and it depends on this property, that the logarithm of any number in this scale, is 1 less than the number of places or figures contained in that power of the given number whose exponent is 10000000000, or the logarithm of 10, at least as to integer numbers, for they really differ by a fraction, as is shown by Mr. Briggs in his illustrations of these properties, printed at the end of this appendix to the construction of logarithms. I shall here set down one more of these relations, as the manner in which it is expressed is exactly similar to that of fluxions and fluents, and it is this: Of any two numbers, as the greater is to the less, so is the velocity of the increment or decrement of the logarithms at the less, to the velocity of the increment or decrement of the logarithms at the greater: that is, in our modern notation, as $X : Y :: \dot{y}$ to $\dot{x}$, where $\dot{x}$ and $\dot{y}$ are the fluxions of the logarithms of X and Y.

Kepler's Construction of Logarithms.

The logarithms of Briggs and Kepler were both printed the same year, 1624; but as the latter are of the same kind as Napier's, we shall here give this author's construction of them, before proceeding to that of Briggs's. We have already (pa. 31 *et seq.*) described the nature and form of Kepler's logarithms, showing that they are of the same kind as Napier's, but only a little varied in the form of the table. It may also be added, that, in general, the ideas which these two masters had on this subject, were of the same nature: only it was more fully and methodically laid down by Kepler, who expanded, and delivered in a regular science, the hints that were given by the illustrious inventor. The foundation and nature of their methods of construction are also the same, but only a little varied in their modes of applying them. Kepler here, first of any, treats of logarithms in the true and genuine way of the measures of ratios, or proportions*, as he calls them, and that in a very full and scientific manner: and this method of his was afterwards followed and abridged by Mercator, Halley, Cotes, and others, as we shall see in the proper places. Kepler first erects a regular and purely mathematical system of proportions, and the measures of proportions, treated at considerable length in a number of propositions, which are fully and chastely demonstrated by genuine mathematical reasoning, and illustrated by examples in numbers. This part contains and de-

* Kepler almost always uses the term *proportion* instead of *ratio*, which I also shall do in my account of his work, as well as conform in expressions and notations to his other peculiarities. It may also be here remarked, that I observe the same practice in describing the works of other authors, the better to convey the idea of their several methods and style. And this may serve to account for some seeming inequalities in the language of this history.

H

monstrates both the nature and the principles of the structure of logarithms. And in the second part he applies those principles in the actual construction of his table, which contains only 1000 numbers, and their logarithms, in the form as we before described : and in this part he indicates the various contrivances employed in deducing the logarithms of proportions one from another, after a few of the leading ones had been first formed, by the general and more remote principles. He uses the name *logarithms*, given them by the inventor, being the most proper, as expressing the very nature and essence of those artificial numbers, and containing as it were a definition in the very name of them ; but without taking any notice of the inventor, or of the origin of those useful numbers.

As this tract is very curious and important in itself, and is besides very rare and little known, instead of a particular description only, I shall here give a brief translation of both the parts, omitting only the demonstrations of the propositions, and some rather long illustrations of them. The book is dedicated to Philip, landgrave of Hesse, but is without either preface or introduction, and commences immediately with the subject of the first part, which is entitled *The Demonstration of the Structure of Logarithms ;* and the contents of it are as follow :

Postulate 1. That all proportions equal among themselves, by whatever variety of couplets of terms they may be denoted, are measured or expressed by the same quantity.

Axiom 1. If there be any number of quantities of the same kind, the proportion of the extremes is understood to be composed of all the proportions of every adjacent couplet of terms, from the first to the last.

1 *Proposition.* The mean proportional between two terms, divides the proportion of those terms into two equal proportions.

Axiom 2. Of any number of quantities regularly increasing, the means divide the proportion of the extremes into one proportion more than the number of the means.

Postulate 2. That the proportion between any two terms is divisible into any number of parts, until those parts become less than any proposed quantity.

An example of this section is then inserted in a small table, in dividing the proportion which is between 10 and 7 into 1073741824 equal parts, by as many mean proportionals wanting one, namely, by taking the mean proportional between 10 and 7, then the mean between 10 and this mean, and the mean between 10 and the last, and so on for 30 means, or 30 extractions of the square root, the last or 30th of which roots is 9999999966782056900 ; and the 30th power of 2, which is 1073741824, shows into how many parts the proportion between 10 and 7, or between 1000&c, and 700&c, is divided by 1073741824 means, each of which parts is equal to the proportion between 1000&c, and the 30th mean 999&c, that is, the proportion between 1000&c, and 999&c, is the 1073741824th part of the proportion between 10 and 7. Then by assuming the small difference 00000000033217943100, for the measure of the very small element of the proportion of 10 to 7, or for the measure of the proportion of 1000&c, to 999&c, or for the logarithm of this last term, and multiplying it by 1073741824, the number of parts, the product gives 35667.49461.37222.14400, for the logarithm of the less term 7 or 700&c.

Postulate 3. That the extremely small quantity or element of a proportion may be measured or denoted by any quantity whatever; as, for instance, by the difference of the terms of that element.

2 *Proposition*. Of three continued proportionals, the difference of the two first has to the difference of the latter two, the same proportion which the first term has to the 2d, or the 2d to the 3d.

3 *Prop*. Of any continued proportionals, the greatest terms have the greatest difference, and the least terms the least.

4 *Prop*. In any continued proportionals, if the difference of the greatest terms be made the measure of the proportion between *them*, the difference of any other couplet will be less than the true measure of *their* proportion.

5 *Prop*. In continued proportionals, if the difference of the greatest terms be made the measure of their proportion, then the measure of the proportion of the greatest to any other term will be greater than *their* difference.

6 *Prop*. In continued proportionals, if the difference of the greatest term and any one of the less, taken not immediately next to it, be made the measure of their proportion, then the proportion which is between the greatest and any other term greater than the one before taken, will be less than the difference of those terms; but the proportion which is between the greatest term, and any one less than that first taken, will be greater than their difference.

7 *Prop*. Of any quantities placed according to the order of their magnitudes, if any two successive proportions be equal, the three successive terms which constitute them will be continued proportionals.

8 *Prop*. Of any quantities placed in the order of their magnitudes, if the intermediates lying between any two terms be not among the mean proportionals which can be interposed between the said two terms, then such intermediates do not divide the proportion of those two terms into commensurable proportions.

Besides the demonstrations, as usual, several definitions are here given; as of commensurable proportions, &c.

9 *Prop*. When two expressible lengths are not to one another as two figurate numbers of the same species, such as two squares, or two cubes, there cannot fall between them other expressible lengths, which shall be mean proportionals, and as many in number as that species requires, namely, one in the squares, two in the cubes, three in the biquadrats, &c.

10 *Prop*. Of any expressible quantities, following in the order of their magnitudes, if the two extremes be not in the proportion of two square numbers, or two cubes, or two other powers of the same kind, none of the intermediates divide the proportion into commensurables.

11 *Prop*. All the proportions, taken in order, which are between expressible terms that are in arithmetical proportion, are incommensurable to one another. As between 8, 13, 18.

12 *Prop*. Of any quantities placed in the order of their magnitude, if

the difference of the greatest terms be made the measure of their proportion, then the difference between any two others will be less than the measure of *their* proportion; and if the difference of the two least terms be made the measure of their proportion, then the differences of the rest will be greater than the measure of the proportion between *their* terms.

Corol. If the measure of the proportion between the greatest exceed their difference, then the proportion of this measure to the said difference, will be less than that of a following measure to the difference of its terms. Because proportionals have the same ratio.

13 *Prop.* If three quantities follow one another in the order of magnitude, the proportion of the two last will be contained in the proportion of the extremes, a less number of times than the difference of the two least is contained in the difference of the extremes: And, on the contrary, the proportion of the two greatest will be contained in the proportion of the extremes, oftener than the difference of the former is contained in that of the latter.

Corol. Hence, if the difference of the two greater be equal to the difference of the two less terms, the proportion between the two greater will be less than the proportion between the two less.

14 *Prop.* Of three equidifferent quantities, taken in order, the proportion between the extremes is more than double the proportion between the two greater terms.

Corol. Hence it follows, that half the proportion of the extremes is greater than the proportion of the two greatest terms, but less than the proportion of the two least.

15 *Prop.* If two quantities constitute a proportion, and each quantity be lessened by half the greater, the remainders will constitute a proportion greater than double the former.

16 *Prop.* The aliquot parts of incommensurable proportions are incommensurable to each other.

17 *Prop.* If one thousand numbers follow one another in the natural order, beginning at 1000, and differing all by unity, viz. 1000, 999, 998, 997,&c; and the proportion between the two greatest 1000, 999, by continual bisection, be cut into parts that are smaller than the excess of the proportion between the next two 999, 998, over the said proportion between the two greatest 1000, 999; and then for the measure of that small element of the proportion between 1000 and 999, there be taken the difference of 1000 and that mean proportional which is the other term of the element. Again, if the proportion between 1000 and 998 be likewise cut into double the number of parts which the former proportion, between 1000 and 999, was cut into: and then for the measure of the small element in this division, be taken the difference of its terms, of which the greater is 1000. And in the same manner, if the proportion of 1000 to the following numbers, as 997, &c, by continual bisection, be cut into particles of such magnitude, as may be between $\frac{3}{4}$ and $\frac{3}{4}$ of the element arising from the section of the first proportion between 1000 and 999, the measure

of each element will be given from the difference of its terms. Then, this being done, the measure of any one of the 1000 proportions will be composed of as many measures of its element as there are of those elements in the said divided proportion. And all these measures, for all the proportions, will be sufficiently exact for the nicest calculations.

All these sections and measures of proportions are performed in the manner of that described at postulate 2, and the operation is abundantly explained by numerical calculations.

18 *Prop.* The proportion of any number, to the first term 1000, being known : there will also be known the proportion of the rest of the numbers in the same continued proportion, to the said first term.

So from the known proportion between 1000 and 900,
there is also known the proportion of 1000 to 810, and to 729 ;
And from 1000 to 800, also 1000 to 640, and to 512 ;
And from 1000 to 700, also 1000 to 490, and to 343 ;
And from 1000 to 600, also 1000 to 360, and to 216 ;
And from 1000 to 500, also 1000 to 250, and to 125.

Corol. Hence arises the precept for squaring, cubing, &c ; as also for extracting the square root, cube root, &c, out of the first figures of numbers. For it will be, as the greatest number of the chiliad, as a denominator, is to the number proposed as a numerator, so is this to the square of the fraction, and so is this to the cube.

19 *Prop.* The proportion of a number to the first, or 1000, being known; if there be two other numbers in the same proportion to each other, then the proportion of one of these to 1000 being known, there will also be known the proportion of the other to the same 1000.

Corol. 1. Hence from the 15 proportions mentioned in prop. 18, will be known 120 others below 1000, to the same 1000.

For so many are the proportions, equal to some one or other of the said 15, that are among the other integer numbers which are less than 1000.

Corol. 2. Hence arises the method of treating the Rule-of-Three, when 1000 is one of the given terms.

For this is effected by adding to, or subtracting from, each other, the measures of the two proportions of 1000 to each of the other two given numbers, according as 1000 is, or is not, the first term in the Rule-of-Three.

20 *Prop.* When four numbers are proportional, the first to the second as the third to the fourth, and the proportions of 1000 to each of the three former are known, there will also be known the proportion of 1000 to the fourth number.

Corol. 1. By this means other chiliads are added to the former.

Corol. 2. Hence arises the method of performing the Rule-of-Three, when 1000 is not one of the terms. Namely, from the sum of the measures of the proportions of 1000 to the second and third, take that of 1000 to the first, and the remainder is the measure of the proportion of 1000 to the fourth term.

Definition. The measure of the proportion between 1000 and any less number as before described, and expressed by a number, is set opposite to that less number in the chiliad, and is called its LOGA-RITHM, that is, the number ($\alpha\rho\iota\vartheta\mu\varsigma$) indicating the proportion ($\lambda\circ\gamma\circ\nu$) which 1000 bears to that number, to which the logarithm is annexed.

21 *Prop.* If the first or greatest number be made the radius of a circle, or sinus totus; every less number, considered as the cosine of some arc, has a logarithm greater than the versed sine of that arc, but less than the difference between the radius and secant of the arc; except only in the term next after the radius, or greatest term, the logarithm of which, by the hypothesis, is made equal to the versed sine.

That is, if CD be made the logarithm of AC, or the measure of the proportion of AC to AD; then the measure of the proportion of AB to AD, that is the logarithm of AB, will be greater than BD, but less than EF. And this is the same as Napier's first rule in page 45.

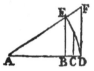

22 *Prop.* The same things being supposed; the sum of the versed sine and excess of the secant over the radius, is greater than double the logarithm of the cosine of an arc.

Corol. The log. cosine is less than the arithmetical mean between the versed sine and the excess of the secant.

Precept 1. Any sine being found in the canon of sines, and its defect below radius to the excess of the secant above radius, then shall the logarithm of the sine be less than half that sum, but greater than the said defect or coversed sine.

Let there be the sine   99970.1490 of an arc:
Its defect below radius is   29.8510 the covers. and less than the log. sine:
Add the excess of the secant 29.8599

             Sum 59.7109
          its half or 29.8555 greater than the logarithm.
Therefore the log. is between 29.8510
            and 29.8555

Precept 2. The logarithm of the sine being found, you will also find nearly the logarithm of the round or integer number, which is next less than the sine with a fraction, by adding that fractional excess to the logarithm of the said sine.

Thus, the logarithm of the sine 99970.149 is found to be about 29.854; if now the logarithm of the round number 99970.000 be required, add 149, the fractional part of the sine, to its logarithm, observing the point, thus,
          29.854
            149

the sum 30.003 is the log. of the round number 99970.000 nearly.

23 *Prop.* Of three equidifferent quantities, the measure of the proportion between the two greater terms, with the measure of the

proportion between the two less terms, will constitute a proportion, which will be greater than the proportion of the two greater terms, but less than the proportion of the two least.

Thus if AB, AC, AD, be three quantities, having the equal differences BC, CD; and if the measure of the proportion of AD, AC be cd, and that of AC, AB be bc; then the proportion of cd to cb will be greater than the proportion of AC to AD, but less than the proportion of AB to AC.

$$\overset{1}{\underset{A}{|}} \quad\quad \overset{1}{\underset{B}{|}} \quad \overset{1}{\underset{C}{|}} \quad \overset{1}{\underset{D}{|}}$$

$$\overset{1}{\underset{b}{|}} \quad \overset{1}{\underset{c}{|}} \quad \overset{1}{\underset{d}{|}}$$

24 *Prop.* The said proportion between the two measures is less than half the proportion between the extreme terms. That is, the proportion between bc, cd, is less than half the proportion between AB, AD.

Corol. Since therefore the arithmetical mean divides the proportion into unequal parts, of which the one is greater, and the other less, than half the whole; if it be inquired what proportion is between these proportions, the answer is, that it is a little less than the said half.

An Example of finding nearly the limits, greater and less, to the measure of any proposed proportion.

It being known that the measure of the proportion between 1000 and 900 is 10536.05, required the measure of the proportion 900 to 800, where the terms 1000, 900, 800, have equal differences. Therefore as 9 to 10, so 10536.05 to 11706.72, which is less than 11778.30 the measure of the proportion 9 to 8. Again, as the mean proportional between 8 and 10 (which is 8.9442719) is to 10, so 10536.05 to 11779.66, which is greater than the measure of the proportion between 9 and 8.

Axiom. Every number denotes an expressible quantity.

25 *Prop.* If the 1000 numbers differing by 1, follow one another in the natural order; and there be taken any two adjacent numbers, as the terms of some proportion; the measure of this proportion will be to the measure of the proportion between the two greatest terms of the chiliad, in a proportion greater than that which the greatest term 1000 bears to the greater of the two terms first taken, but less than the proportion of 1000 to the less of the said two selected terms.

So, of the 1000 numbers, taking any two successive terms, as 501 and 500, the logarithm of the former being 69114.92, and of the latter 69314.72, the difference of which is 199.80. Therefore, by the definition, the measure of the proportion between 501 and 500 is 199.80. In like manner, because the logarithm of the greatest term 1000 is 0, and of the next 999 is 100.05, the difference of these logarithms, and the measure of the proportion between 1000 and 999, is 100.05. Couple now the greatest term 1000 with each of the selected terms 501 and 500; couple also the measure 199.80 with the measure 100.05; so shall the proportion between 199.80 and 100.05, be greater than the proportion between 1000 and 501, but less than the proportion between 1000 and 500.

Corol. 1. Any number below the first 1000 being proposed, as also its logarithm, the differences of any logarithms antecedent to that proposed, towards the beginning of the chiliad, are to the first logarithm (viz. that which is assigned to 999) in a greater proportion than 1000 to the number proposed; but of those which follow towards the last logarithm, they are to the same in a less proportion.

Corol. 2. By this means, the places of the chiliad may easily be filled up, which have not yet had logarithms adapted to them by the former propositions.

26 *Prop.* The difference of two logarithms, adapted to two adjacent numbers, is to the difference of these numbers, in a proportion greater than 1000 bears to the greater of those numbers, but less than that of 1000 to the less of the two numbers.

This 26th prop. is the same as Napier's second rule, at page 45.

27 *Prop.* Having given two adjacent numbers, of the 1000 natural numbers, with their logarithmic indices, or the measures of the proportions which those absolute or round numbers constitute with 1000, the greatest; the increments, or differences, of these logarithms, will be to the logarithm of the small element of the proportions, as the secants of the arcs whose cosines are the two absolute numbers, is to the greatest number, or the radius of the circle; so that, however, of the said two secants, the less will have to the radius a less proportion than the proposed difference has to the first of all, but the greater will have a greater proportion, and so also will the mean proportional between the said secants have a greater proportion.

Thus if BC, CD be equal, also b d the logarithm of A B, and c d the logarithm of A C; then the proportion of b c to c d will be greater than the proportion of A G to A D, but less than that of A F to A D, and also less than that of the mean proportional between A F and A G to A D.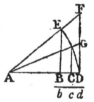

Corol. 1. The same obtains also when the two terms differ, not only by the unit of the small element, but by another unit, which may be ten fold, a hundred fold, or a thousand fold of that.

Corol. 2. Hence the differences will be obtained sufficiently exact, especially when the absolute numbers are pretty large, by taking the arithmetical mean between two small secants, or (if you will be at the labour) by taking the geometrical mean between two larger secants, and then by continually adding the differences, the logarithms will be produced.

Corol. 3. *Precept.* Divide the radius by each term of the assigned proportion, and the arithmetical mean (or still nearer the geometrical mean) between the quotients, will be the required increment; which being added to the logarithm of the greater term, will give the logarithm of the less term.

Example.

Let there be given the logarithm of 700, viz. 35667.4948, to find the log. to 699.
Here radius divided by 700 gives 1428571 &c.
and divided by 699 gives 1430672 &c.
the arithmetic. mean is 142.962
which added to 35667.4948

gives the logarithm to 699   35810.4568

Corol. 4. *Precept* for the logarithms of sines.
The increment between the logarithms of two sines, is thus found: find the geometrical mean between the cosecants, and divide it by the difference of the sines, the quotient will be the difference of the logarithms.

Example.

0° 1′ sine 2909   cosec. 343774682 | The quotient 80000 exceeds the re-
0 2 sine 5818   cosec. 171887319 | quired increment of the logarithms, be-
                      | cause the secants are here so large.
dif. 2909 geom. mean 2428 nearly.

Appendix. Nearly in the same manner it may be shown, that the second differences are in the duplicate proportion of the first, and the third in the duplicate of the second. Thus, for instance, in the beginning of the logarithms, the first difference is 100.00000, viz. equal to the difference of the numbers 100000.00000 and 99900.00000; the second or difference of the differences, 10000; the third 20. Again, after arriving at the number 50000.00000, the logarithms have for a difference 200.00000, which is to the first difference, as the number 100000.00000 to 50000.00000; but the second difference is 40000, in which 10000 is contained 4 times; and the third 328, in which 20 is contained 16 times. But since in treating of new matters we labour under the want of proper words, therefore, lest we should become too obscure, the demonstration is omitted untried.

28 *Prop.* No number expresses exactly the measure of the proportion between two of the 1000 numbers, constituted by the foregoing method.

29 *Prop.* If the measures of all proportions be expressed by numbers or logarithms; all proportions will not have assigned to them their due portion of measure, to the utmost accuracy.

30 *Prop.* If to the number 1000, the greatest of the chiliad, be referred others that are greater than it, and the logarithm of 1000 be made 0, the logarithms belonging to those greater numbers will be negative.

This concludes the first or scientific part of the work, the principles of which Kepler applies, in the second part, to the actual construction of the first 1000 logarithms, which construction is pretty minutely described. This part is entitled *A very compendious Method of constructing the Chiliad of Logarithms;* and it is not improperly so called, the method being very concise and easy. The fundamental principles are briefly these: That at the beginning of the logarithms, their in-

1

crements or differences are equal to those of the natural numbers : that the natural numbers may be considered as the decreasing cosines of increasing arcs; and that the secants of those arcs at the beginning have the same differences as the cosines, and therefore the same differences as the logarithms. Then, since the secants are the reciprocals of the cosines, by these principles and the third corollary to the 27th proposition, he establishes the following method of constituting the 100 first or smallest logarithms to the 100 largest numbers, 1000, 999, 998, 997, &c, to 900. viz. Divide the radius 1000, increased with seven ciphers, by each of these numbers separately, disposing the quotients in a table, and they will be the secants of those arcs which have the divisors for their cosines; continuing the division to the 8th figure, as it is in that place only that the arithmetical and geometrical means differ. Then by adding successively the arithmetical means between every two successive secants, the sums will be the series of logarithms. Or by adding continually every two secants, the successive sums will be the series of the double logarithms.

Besides these 100 logarithms, thus constructed, he constitutes two others by continual bisection, or extractions of the square root, after the manner described in the second postulate. And first he finds the logarithm which measures the proportion between 100000.00 and 97656.25, which latter term is the third proportional to 1024 and 1000, each with two ciphers; and this is effected by means of twenty-four continual extractions of the square root, determining the greatest term of each of twenty-four classes of mean proportionals; then the difference between the greatest of these means and the first or whole number 1000, with ciphers, being as often doubled, there arises 2371.6526 for the logarithm sought, which made negative is the logarithm of 1024. Secondly, the like process is repeated for the proportion between the numbers 1000 and 500, from which arises 69314.7193 for the logarithm of 500; which he also calls the logarithm of duplication, being the measure of the proportion of 2 to 1.

Then from the foregoing he derives all the other logarithms in the chiliad, beginning with those of the prime numbers 1, 2, 3, 5, 7, &c, in the first 100. And first, since 1024, 512, 256, 128, 64, 32, 16, 8, 4, 2, 1, are all in the continued proportion of 1000 to 500, therefore the proportion of 1024 to 1 is decuple of the proportion of 1000 to 500, and consequently the logarithm of 1 would be decuple of the logarithm of 500, if 0 were taken as the logarithm of 1024; but since the logarithm of 1024 is applied negatively, the logarithm of 1 must be diminished by as much : diminishing therefore 10 times the logarithm of 500, which is 693147.1928, by 2371.6526, the remainder 690775.5422 is the logarithm of 1, or of 100.00, what is set down in the table.

And because 1, 10, 100, 1000, are continued proportionals, therefore the proportion of 1000 to 1 is triple of the proportion of 1000 to 100, and consequently $\frac{1}{3}$ of the logarithm of 1 is to be put for the logarithm of 100, viz. 230258.5141, and this is also the logarithm of decuplication, or of the pro-

Nos.	Logarithms.
100	230258.5141
10	460517.0282
1	690775.5423
.1	921034.0563
.01	1151292.5703
.001	1381551.0844
.0001	1611809.5965

portion of 10 to 1. And hence, multiplying this logarithm of 100 successively by 2, 3, 4, 5, 6, and 7, there arise the logarithms to the numbers in the decuple proportion, as in the margin.

Also if the logarithm of duplication, or of the proportion of 2 to 1, be taken from the logarithm of 1, there will remain the logarithm of 2; and from the logarithm of 2 taking the logarithm of 10, there remains the logarithm of the proportion of 5 to 1; which taken from the logarithm of 1, there remains the logarithm of 5. See the margin.

Log. of 1	690775.5422
of 2 to 1	693l4.7193
log. of 2	621460.8229
log. of 10	460517.0281
of 5 to 1	160943.7948
log. of 5	529831.7474

For the logarithms of other prime numbers, he has recourse to those of some of the first or greatest century of numbers, before found, viz. of 999, 998, 997, &c. And first, taking 960, whose logarithm is 4082.2001; then by adding to this logarithm the logarithm of duplication, there will arise the several logarithms of all those numbers, which are in duplicate proportion continued from 960, namely 480, 240, 120, 60, 30, 15. Hence, the logarithm of 30 taken from the logarithm of 10, leaves the logarithm of the proportion of 3 to 1; which taken from the logarithm of 1, leaves the logarithm of 3, viz. 580914.3106. And the double of this diminished by the logarithm of 1, gives 471053.0790 for the logarithm of 9.

Next, from the logarithm of 990, or 9 × 10 × 11, which is 1005.0331, he finds the logarithm of 11, namely, subtract the sum of the logarithms of 9 and 10 from the sum of the logarithm of 990 and double the logarithm of 1, there remains 450986.0106 the logarithm of 11.

Again, from the logarithm of 980, or 2 × 10 × 7 × 7, which is 2020.2711, he finds 496184.5228 for the logarithm of 7.

And from 5129.3303 the logarithm of 950, or 5 × 10 × 19, he finds 396331.6392 for the logarithm of 19.

In like manner the logarithm

to 998 or 4 × 13 × 19, gives the logarithm of 13;
to 969 or 3 × 17 × 19, gives the logarithm of 17;
to 986 or 2 × 17 × 29, gives the logarithm of 29;
to 966 or 6 × 7 × 23, gives the logarithm of 23;
to 930 or 3 × 10 × 31, gives the logarithm of 31.

And so on for all the primes below 100, and for many of the primes in the other centuries up to 900. After which, he directs to find the logarithms of all numbers composed of these, by the proper addition and subtraction of their logarithms, namely, in finding the logarithm of the product of two numbers, from the sum of the logarithms of the two factors take the logarithm of 1, the remainder is the logarithm of the product. In this way he shows that the logarithms of all numbers under 500 may be derived, except those of the following 36 numbers, namely, 127, 149, 167, 173, 179, 211, 223, 251, 257, 263, 269, 271, 277, 281, 283, 293, 337, 347, 349, 353, 359, 367, 373, 379, 383, 389, 397, 401, 409, 419, 421, 431, 433, 439, 443, 449. Also, besides the composite numbers between 500 and 900, made up of the products of some numbers whose logarithms have been before determined, there will be 59 primes not composed of them; which, with the 36 above mentioned, make 95 numbers in all, not composed of the products of any before them, and the logarithms of which he directs to be derived in this manner; namely, by considering the differences of the logarithms of the numbers interspersed among them: then by that method by which were constituted the differences of the logarithms of the smallest 100 numbers in a continued series, we are to proceed here in the discontinued series, that is, by prop. 27, corol. 3, and especially by the appendix to it, if it be rightly used, whence those differences will be very easily supplied.

This closes the second part, or the actual construction of the logarithms; after which follows the table itself, which has been before described, pa. 32. Before dismissing Kepler's work, however, it may not be improper in this place to take notice of an erroneous property laid down by him in the appendix to the 27th prop. just now referred to; both because it is an error in principle, tending to vitiate the practice, and because it serves to show that Kepler was unacquainted with the true nature of the orders of differences of the logarithms, notwithstanding what he says above with respect to the construction of them by means of their several orders of differences, and that consequently he has no legal claim to any share in the discovery of the differential method, known at that time to Briggs, and it would seem to him alone, it being published in his logarithms in the same year, 1624, as Kepler's book, together with the true nature of the logarithmic orders of differences, as we shall presently see in the following account of his works. Now this error of Kepler's here alluded to, is in that expression where he says the third differences are in the *duplicate* ratio of the second differences, like as the second differences are in the duplicate ratio of the first; or, in other words, that the third differences are as the *squares* of the second differences, as well as the second differences as the squares of the first; or that the third differences are as the *fourth powers* of the first differences. Whereas in truth the third differences are only as the *cubes* of the first differences. Kepler seems to have been led into this error by a mistake in his numbers, viz. when he says in that appendix, that the *third difference is* 328, *in which* 20 *is contained* 16 *times;* for when the numbers are accurately computed, the third difference comes out only 161, in which therefore 20 is contained only 8 times, which is the cube of 2, the number of times the one first difference contains the other. It would hence seem that Kepler had hastily drawn the above erroneous principle from this one numerical example, or little more, false as it is: for had he made the trial in many instances, though erroneously computed, they could not easily have been so uniformly so, as to afford the same false conclusion. And therefore from hence, and what he says at the conclusion of that appendix, it may be inferred, that he either never attempted the demonstration of the property in question, or else that he found himself embarrassed with it, and unable to accomplish it, and therefore dispatched it in the ambiguous manner in which it appears.

But it may easily be shown, not only that the third differences of the logarithms at different places, are as the cubes of the first differences; but, in general, that the numbers in any one and the same order of differences, at different places, are as that power of the numbers in the first differences, whose index is the same as that of the order : or that the second, third, fourth, &c, differences, will be as the second, third, fourth, &c, powers of the first differences. For the several orders of differences, when the absolute numbers differ by indefinitely small parts, are as the several orders of fluxions of the logarithms; but if

x be any number, then $\dfrac{m\dot{x}}{x}$ is the fluxion of the logarithm of x, to the modulus m, and the second fluxion, or the fluxion of this fluxion,

is $-\dfrac{m\dot{x}^2}{x^2}$, since $\dot{x}$ is constant: and the third, fourth, &c, fluxions

are $\dfrac{2m\dot{x}^3}{x^3}$, $-\dfrac{2.3m\dot{x}^4}{x^4}$, &c; that is, the first, second, third, fourth, fifth, sixth, &c, orders of fluxions, are equal to the modulus m multiplied into each of these terms,

$$\frac{\dot{x}}{x}, \quad -\frac{1\dot{x}^2}{x^2}, \quad \frac{1.2\dot{x}^3}{x^3}, \quad -\frac{1.2.3\dot{x}^4}{x^4}, \quad \frac{1.2.3.4\dot{x}^5}{x^5}, \quad -\frac{1.2.3.4.5\dot{x}^6}{x^6}, \&c;$$

where it is evident, that the fluxion of any order is as that power of the first fluxion, whose index is the same as the number of the order. And these quantities would actually be the several terms of the differences themselves, if the differences of the numbers were indefinitely small. But they vary the more from them, as the differences of the absolute numbers differ from $\dot{x}$, or as the said constant numerical difference 1 approaches towards the value of x the number itself. However, on the whole, the several orders vary proportionably, so as still sensibly to preserve the same analogy, namely, that two nth differences are in proportion as the nth powers of their respective first differences.

Of Briggs's Construction of his Logarithms.

Nearly according to the methods described in page 48, Mr. Briggs constructed the logarithms of the prime numbers, as appears from his relation of this business in the *Arithmetica Logarithmica*, printed in 1624, where he details, in an ample manner, the whole construction and use of his logarithms. The work is divided into 32 chapters or sections. In the first of these, logarithms in a general sense are defined, and some properties of them illustrated. In the second chapter he remarks, that it is most convenient to make 0 the logarithm of 1; and on that supposition he exemplifies these following properties, namely, that the logarithms of all numbers are either the indices of powers, or proportional to them; that the sum of the logarithms of two or more factors, is the logarithm of their product; and that the difference of the logarithms of two numbers, is the logarithm of their quotient. In the third section, he states the other assumption which is necessary to limit his system of logarithms, namely, making 1 the logarithm of 10, as that which produces the most convenient form of logarithms : He hence also takes occasion to show that the powers of 10, namely, 100, 1000, &c, are the only numbers which can have rational logarithms. The fourth section treats of the characteristic ; by which name he distinguishes the integral, or first part, of a logarithm towards the left hand, which expresses 1 less than the number of integer places or figures in the number belonging to that logarithm, or how far the first figure of this number is removed from the place of units ; namely, that 0 is the characteristic of the logarithms of all numbers from 1 to 10 ; and 1 the characteristic of all those from 10 to 100 ; and 2 that of those from 100 to 1000 ; and so on.

He begins the fifth chapter with remarking, that his logarithms may chiefly be constructed by the two methods which were mentioned by Napier, as above related, and for the sake of which he here premises several *lemmata*, concerning the powers of numbers and their indices, and how many places of figures are in the products of numbers, observing that the product of two numbers will consist of as many figures as there are in both factors, unless perhaps the product of the first figures in each factor be expressed by one figure only, which often happens, and then commonly there will be 1 figure in the product less than in the two factors ; as also that, of any two of the terms in a series of geometricals, the results will be equal by raising each term to the power denoted by the index of the other ; or any number raised to the power denoted by the logarithm of the other, will be equal to this latter number raised to the power denoted by the logarithm of the former ; and consequently if the one number be 10, whose logarithm is one with any number of ciphers, then any number raised to the power whose index is 1000 &c, or the logarithm of 10, will be equal to 10 raised to the power whose index is the logarithm of that number ; that is, the logarithm of any number in this scale, where 1 is the logarithm of 10, is the index of that power of 10 which is equal to the given number. But the index of any integral power of 10, is 1 less than the number of places in that power, consequently the logarithm of any other number, which is no integral power of 10, is not quite one less than the number of places in that power of the given number whose index is 1000 &c, or the logarithm of 10.

Find therefore the 10th, or 100th, or 1000th, &c, power of any number, as suppose 2, with the number of figures in such power ; then shall that number of figures always exceed the logarithm of 2, though the excess will be constantly less than 1.

An example of this process is here given in the margin; where the 1st column contains the several powers of 2, the 2d their corresponding indices, and the 3d contains the number of places in the powers in the first column; and of these numbers in the third column, such as are on the lines of those indices that consist of 1 with ciphers, are continual approximations to the logarithm of 2, being always too great by less than 1 in the last figure, that logarithm being 3.0102999566398 &c.

And here, since the exact powers of 2 are not required, but only the number of figures they consist of, as shown by the third column, only a few of the first figures of the powers in the first column are retained, those being sufficient to determine the number of places in them; and the multiplications in raising these powers are performed in a contracted way, so as to have the fifth or last figure in them true to the nearest unit. Indeed these multiplications might be performed in the same manner, retaining only the first three figures, and those to the nearest unit in the third place; which would make this a very easy way indeed of finding the logarithms of a few prime numbers.

Powers of 2	Indices.	No. of places or logs.
2	1	1
4	2	1
16	4	2
256	8	3
1024	10	4 log. of 2
10486	20	7 log. of 4
10995	40	13 log. of 16
12089	80	25 log. of 256
12676	100	31 log. of 2
16069	200	61 log. of 4
25823	400	121 log. 16
66680	800	241 log. 256
10715	1000	302 log. 2
11481	2000	603 log. 4
13182	4000	1205 log. 16
17377	8000	2409 log. 256
19950	10000	3011 log. 2
39803	20000	6021 log. 4
15843	40000	12042 log. 16
25099	80000	24083 log. 256
99900	100000	30103 log. 2
99801	200000	60206 log. 4
99601	400000	120412 &c.
99204	800000	240824
99006	1000000	301030
98023	2000000	602060
96085	4000000	1204120
92323	8000000	2408240
90498	10000000	3010300
81899	20000000	6020600
67075	40000000	12041200
44990	80000000	24082400
36846	100000000	30103000
13577	200000000	60206000
18433	400000000	120411999
33977	800000000	240823997
46129	1000000000	301029996

It may also be remarked, that those several powers, whose indices are 1 with ciphers, are raised by thrice squaring from the former powers, and multiplying the first by the third of these squares; making also the corresponding doublings and additions of their indices: thus, the square of 2 is 4, and the square of 4 is 16, the square of 16 is 256, and 256 multiplied by 4 is 1024; in like manner, the double of 1 is 2, the double of 2 is 4, the double of 4 is 8, and 8 added to 2 makes 10. And the same for all the following powers and indices. The numbers in the third column, which show how many places are in the corresponding powers in the first column, are produced in the very same way as those in the second column, namely, by three duplications and one addition; only observing to subtract 1 when the product of the first figures are expressed by one figure, or when the first figures exceed those of the number or power next above them. It may further be observed, that, like as the first number in each quaternion, or space of four lines or numbers, in the third column, approximates to the logarithm of 2, the first number in the first quaternion of the first column; so the second, third, and fourth terms of each quaternion in the third column, approximate to the logarithm of 4, 16, and 256, the second, third, and fourth numbers in the first quaternion in the first column. And moreover, by cutting off one, two, three, &c, figures, as the index or integral part, from the said logarithms of 2, 4, 16, and 256, the first, second, third, and fourth numbers in the first quaternion of the first column, the remaining figures will be the decimal part of the logarithms of the corresponding first, second, third, and fourth numbers in the following second, third, fourth, &c, quaternions: the reason of which is, that any number of any quaternion in the first column, is the tenth power of the corresponding term in the next preceding quaternion. So that the third column contains the logarithms of all the numbers in the first column: a property which if Dr. Newton had been aware of, he could not well have committed such gross mistakes as are found in a table of his similar to that above given, in which most of the numbers in the latter quaternions are totally erroneous; and his confused and imperfect account of this method would induce one to believe that he did not well understand it.

In the 6th chapter our illustrious author begins to treat of the other general method of finding the logarithms of prime numbers, which he thinks an easier way than the former, at least when the logarithm is required to a great many places of figures. This method consists in taking a great number of continued geometrical means between 1 and the given number, whose logarithm is required; that is, first extracting the square root of the given number, then the root of the first root, the root of the second root, the root of the third root, and so on till the last root shall exceed 1 by a very small decimal, greater or less according to the intended number of places to be in the logarithm sought: then finding the logarithm of this small number, by methods described below, he doubles it as often as he made extractions of the square root, or, which is the same thing, he multiplies it by such power of 2 as is denoted by the said number of extractions, and the result is the required logarithm of the given number; as is evident from the nature of logarithms. The rule to know how far to continue this extraction of roots is, that the number of decimal places in the last root be double the number of true places required to be found in the logarithm, and that the first half of them be ciphers; the integer being 1: the reason of which is, that then the significant figures in the decimal, after the ciphers, are directly proportional to those in the corresponding logarithms; such figures in the natural number being the half of those in the next preceding number, like as the logarithm of the last number is the half of the preceding logarithm. Therefore any one such small number, with its logarithm, being once found by the continual extractions of square roots out of a given number, as 10, and corresponding bisections of its given logarithm 1; the logarithm for any other such small number, derived by like continual extractions from another given number, whose logarithm is sought, will be found by one single proportion: which logarithm is then to be doubled according to the number of extractions, or multiplied at once by the like power of 2, for the logarithm of the number proposed. To find the first small number and its logarithm, our author begins with the number 10 and its logarithm 1, and extracts continually the root of the last number and bisects its logarithm, as here registered in the margin, but to far more places of figures, till he arrives at the 53d and 54th roots, with their annexed logarithms, as here below:

	10, given no.	1, its log.
1	3·162277 &c.	0·5
2	1·778279	0·25
3	1·333521	0·125
4	1·154781	0·0625
5	1 074607	0·03125
	&c.	&c.

Numbers. Logarithms.

53|1·00000,00000,00000,25563,82986,40064,70|0·00000,00000,00000.11102,23024,62515.65404
54|1·00000,00000,00000,12781,91493,20632,35|0·00000,00000,00000,05551,11512,31257,82702

where the decimals in the natural numbers are to each other in the ratio of the logarithms, namely, in the ratio of 2 to 1: and therefore any other such small number being found, by continual extraction or otherwise, it will then be as 12781, &c, is to 5551 &c, so is that other small decimal, to the corresponding significant figures of its logarithm. But as every repetition of this proportion requires both a very long multiplication and division, he reduces this constant ratio to another equivalent ratio whose antecedent is 1, by which all the divisions are saved: thus,

as 12781 &c : 5551 &c : : 1000 &c : 434294481903251804,

that is, the logarithm of 1·00000,00000,00000,1

is 0·00000,00000,00000,04342,94481,90325,1804;

and therefore this last number being multiplied by any such small decimal, found as above by continual extraction, the product will be the corresponding logarithm of such last root.

But as the extraction of so many roots is a very troublesome operation, our author devises some ingenious contrivances to abridge that labour. And first, in the 7th chapter, by the following device, to have fewer and easier extractions to perform: namely, raising the powers from any given prime number, whose logarithm is sought, till a power of it be found such that its first figure on the left hand is 1, and the next to it either one or more ciphers; then, having divided this power by 1 with as many ciphers as it has figures after the first, or supposing all after the first to be decimals, the continual roots from this power are extracted till the decimal become sufficiently small, as when the first fifteen places are ciphers; and then by multiplying the decimal by 43429 &c, he has the logarithm of this last root; which logarithm multiplied by the like power of the number 2,

K

gives the logarithm of the first number from which the extraction was begun: to this logarithm prefixing a 1, or 2, or 3, &c, according as this number was found by dividing the power of the given prime number by 10, or 100, or 1000, &c; and lastly, dividing the result by the index of that power, the quotient will be the required logarithm of the given prime number. Thus, to find the logarithm of 2: it is first raised to the 10th power, as in the margin, before the first figures come to be 10; then, dividing by 1000, or cutting off for decimals all the figures after the first or 1, the root is continually extracted out of the quotient 1,024, till the 47th extraction, which gives 1,00000,00000,00000,16851,60570,53949,77; the decimal part of which multiplied by 43429&c, gives 0,00000,00000,00000,07318,55936,90623,9368 for its logarithm; and this being continually doubled for 47 times, gives the logarithms of all the roots up to the first number: or being at once multiplied by the 47th power of 2, viz. 140737488355328, which is raised as in the margin, it gives 0,01029,99566,39811,95265,27744 for the logarithm of the number 1,024, true to 17 or 18 decimals: to this prefix 3, so shall 3,0102 &c be the logarithm of 1024: and lastly, because 2 is the tenth root of 1024, divide by 10, so shall 0,30102,99956,63981,1952 be the logarithm required to the given number 2.

2	1
4	2
8	3
16	4
32	5
64	6
128	7
256	8
512	9
1024	10

2	1
4	2
8	3
16	4
32	5
64	6
128	7
256	8
512	9
1024	10
1048576	20
1073741824	30
1099511627776	40
140737488355328	47

The logarithms of 1, 2, and 10 being now known; it is remarked that the logarithm of 5 becomes known; for since 10÷2 is = 5, the refore log. 10 — log. 2 = log. 5, which is 0,69897,00043,36018,3058; and that from the multiplications and divisions of these three, 2, 5, 10, with the corresponding additions and subtractions of their logarithms, a multitude of other numbers and their logarithms are produced; so, from the powers of 2 are obtained 4, 8, 16, 32, 64, &c; from the powers of 5, these, 25, 125, 625, 3125, &c; also the powers of 5 by those of 10 give 250, 1250, 6250, &c; and the powers of 2 by those of 10, give 20, 200, 2000, &c; 40, 400, 80, 800, &c; likewise by division are obtained 2¼, 1¼, 12½, 6¼, 1½, 3½, 6⅓, &c.

Briggs then observes, that the logarithm of 3, the next prime number, will be best derived from that of 6, in this manner: 6 raised to the 9th power becomes 10077696, which divided by 10000000, gives 1,0077696, and the root from this continually extracted till the 46th, is 1,00000,00000,00000,10998,59345,88155,71866; the decimal part of which multiplied by 43429&c, gives 0,00000,00000,00000,04776,62844,78608,0304 for its logarithm; and this 46 times doubled, or multiplied by the 46th power of 2, gives 0,00336,12534,52792,69 for the logarithm of 1,0077696: to which adding 7, the logarithm of the divisor 10000000, and dividing by 9, the index of the power of 6, there results 0,77815,12503,83643,63 for the logarithm of 6; from which subtracting the logarithm of 2, there remains 0,47712,12547,19662,44 for the logarithm of 3.

In the 8th chapter our ingenious author describes an original and easy method of constructing, by means of differences, the continual mean proportionals which were before found by the extraction of roots. And this, with the other methods of generating logarithms by differences, in this book as well as in his *Trigonometria Britannica*, are I believe the first instances that are to be found of making such use of differences, and show that he was the inventor of what may be called the *Differential Method*. He seems to have discovered this method in the following manner: having observed that these continual means between 1 and any number proposed, found by the continual extraction of roots, approach always nearer and nearer to the halves of each preceding root, as is visible when they are placed together under each other; and indeed it is found that as many of the significant figures of each decimal part, as there are ciphers between them and the integer 1, agree with the half of those above them; I say, having observed this evident approximation, he subtracted each of these decimal parts, which he called A or the first differences, from half the next preceding one, and by comparing together the remainders or second differences, called B, he found that the succeeding were always nearly equal to $\frac{1}{4}$ of the next preceding ones; then taking the difference between each second difference and $\frac{1}{4}$ of the preceding one, he found that these third differences, called C, were nearly in the continual ratio of 8 to 1; again taking the difference between each C and $\frac{1}{4}$ of the next preceding, he found that these fourth differences, called D, were nearly in the continual ratio of 16 to 1; and so on, the 5th (E), 6th (F), &c, differences, being nearly in the continual ratio of 32 to 1, of 64 to 1, &c.

These plain observations being made, they very naturally and clearly suggested to him the notion and method of constructing all the remaining numbers from the differences of a few of the first, found by extracting the roots in the usual way. This will evidently appear from the annexed specimen of a few of the first numbers in the last example for finding the logarithm of 6; where, after the 9th number the rest are supposed to be constructed from the preceding differences of each, as here shown in the 10th and 11th. And it is evident, that in proceeding, the trouble will become always less and less, the differences gradually vanishing, till at last only the first differences remain; and that generally each less difference is shorter than the next greater, by as many places as there are ciphers at the beginning of the decimal in the number to be generated from the differences.

		1,00776,96	
1		1,00387,72833,36962,45663,84655,1	
2		1,00193,67661,36946,61675,87022,9	
3		1,00096,79146,39099,01728,89072,0	
4		1,00048,38402,68846,62985,49253,5	A
5		1,00024,18908,78824,68563,80872,7	A
		24,19201,34423,31492,74626,7	$\frac{1}{2}$A
		292,55598,62978,93754,0	B
6		1,00012,09381,26397,13459,43919,4	A
		12,09454,39412,34281,90436,3	$\frac{1}{2}$A
		73,13015,20822,46516,9	B
		73,13899,65732,23438,5	$\frac{1}{4}$B
		884,44909,76921,5	C
7		1,00006,04672,35055,30968,01600,5	A
		6,04690,63198,56729,71959,7	$\frac{1}{2}$A
		18,28143,25761,70359,2	B
		18,28253,80205,61629,2	$\frac{1}{4}$B
		110,54443,91270,0	C
		110,55613,72115,2	$\frac{1}{8}$C
		1169,80845,2	D
8		1,00003,02331,60505,65775,96479,4	A
		3,02336,17527,65484,00800,2	$\frac{1}{2}$A
		4,57021,99708,04320,8	B
		4,57035,81440,42589,8	$\frac{1}{4}$B
		13,81732,38269,0	C
		13,81805,48908,7	$\frac{1}{8}$C
		73,10639,7	D
		73,11302,8	$\frac{1}{16}$D
		663,1	E
9		1,00001,51164,65999,05672,95048,8	A
		1,51165,80252,82887,98239,7	$\frac{1}{2}$A
		1,14253,77215,03190,9	B
	Hitherto the	1,14255,49927,01080,2	$\frac{1}{4}$B
	smaller differences	1,72711,97889,3	C
	are found by sub-	1,72716,54783,6	$\frac{1}{8}$C
	tracting the larger from	4,56894,3	D
	the parts of the like pre-	4,56915,0	$\frac{1}{16}$D
	ceding ones	20,7	E
		20,7	$\frac{1}{32}$E
	Here the greater differences	65	$\frac{1}{32}$E
	remain after subtracting	28555,89	$\frac{1}{16}$D
	the smaller from the parts	28555,24	D
	of the difference of	21588,99736,16	$\frac{1}{8}$C
	the next preceding	21588,71180,92	C
	number.	28563,44303,75797,72	$\frac{1}{4}$B
		28563,22715,04616,80	B
		75582,32999,52836,47524,40	$\frac{1}{2}$A
10		1,00000,75582,04436,30121,42907,60	A
		2	$\frac{1}{32}$E
		1784,70	$\frac{1}{16}$D
		1784,68	D
		2698,58897,62	$\frac{1}{8}$C
		2698,57112,94	C
		7140,80678,76154,20	$\frac{1}{4}$B
		7140,77980,19041,26	B
		37791,02218,15060,71453,80	$\frac{1}{2}$A
11		1,00000,37790,95077,37080,52412,54	A

He then concludes this chapter with an ingenious, but not obvious, method of finding the differences B,C,D,E, &c. belonging to any number, as suppose the 9th, from that number itself, independent of any of the preceding 8th, 7th, 6th, 5th, &c, and it is this: raise the decimal A to the 2d, 3d, 4th, 5th, &c powers; then will the 2d (B), 3d (C), 4th (D), &c differences, be as here below, viz.

$B = \frac{1}{2}A^2$,

$C = \quad \frac{1}{2}A^3 + \frac{1}{4}A^4$,

$D = \quad\quad \frac{7}{8}A^4 + \frac{7}{8}A^5 + \frac{7}{16}A^6 + \quad \frac{1}{8}A^7 + \quad \frac{1}{64}A^8$,

$E = \quad\quad\quad 2\frac{5}{8}A^5 + 7A^6 + 10\frac{11}{16}A^7 + 12\frac{69}{64}A^8 + 11\frac{11}{64}A^9 + \quad 7\frac{105}{128}A^{10}$,

$F = \quad\quad\quad\quad 13\frac{9}{16}A^6 + 81\frac{1}{8}A^7 + 296\frac{87}{128}A^8 + 834\frac{43}{128}A^9 + 1953\frac{211}{512}A^{10}$ &c.

$G = \quad\quad\quad\quad\quad 122\frac{1}{16}A^7 + 1510\frac{67}{128}A^8 + 11475\frac{73}{128}A^9 + 68372\frac{79}{2048}A^{10}$ &c.

$H = \quad\quad\quad\quad\quad\quad 1937\frac{95}{128}A^8 + 47151\frac{93}{128}A^9 + 706845\frac{149\frac{1}{2}}{8192}A^{10}$ &c.

$I = \quad\quad\quad\quad\quad\quad\quad 54902\frac{89}{128}A^9 + 2558465\frac{215\frac{57}{327\cdot 0}}{}A^{10}$ &c.

$K = \quad\quad\quad\quad\quad\quad\quad\quad 2805527A^{10}$ &c.

&c.

Thus in the 9th number of the foregoing example, omitting the ciphers at the beginning of the decimals, we have

$A = 1,51164,65999,05672,95048,8$

$A^2 = \quad\quad 2,28507,54430,06381,6726$

$A^3 = \quad\quad\quad\quad 3,45422,65239,48546,2$

$A^4 = \quad\quad\quad\quad\quad\quad 5,22156,97802,288$

$A^5 = \quad\quad\quad\quad\quad\quad\quad\quad 7,89316,8205$

$A^6 = \quad\quad\quad\quad\quad\quad\quad\quad\quad\quad 11,93168,1$

&c.

Consequently,

$\frac{1}{2}A^2 = 1,14253,77215,03190,8363 \quad = B$

$\frac{1}{2}A^3 - \quad 1,72711,32619,74273$

$\frac{1}{4}A^4 - \quad\quad\quad 65269,62225$

$\frac{1}{2}A^3 + \frac{1}{4}A^4 \quad \overline{1,72711,97889,36498} \quad = C$

$\frac{7}{8}A^4 \quad 4,56887,35577$

$\frac{7}{8}A^5 - \quad\quad 6,90652$

$\frac{7}{16}A^6 - \quad\quad\quad 5$

$\frac{7}{8}A^4 + \frac{7}{8}A^5 + \frac{7}{16}A^6 \quad \overline{4,56894,26234} \quad = D$

$2\frac{5}{8}A^5 - \quad\quad 20,71957$

$7A^6 - \quad\quad\quad 83$

$2\frac{5}{8}A^5 + 7A^6 - \quad\quad\quad \overline{20,72040} \quad = E$

which agree with the like differences in the foregoing specimen.

In the 9th chapter, after observing that from the logarithms of 1, 2, 3, 5, and 10, before found, are to be determined, by addition and subtraction, the logarithms of all other numbers which can be produced from these by multiplication and division; for finding the logarithms of other prime numbers, instead of that in the seventh chapter, our author then shows another ingenious method of obtaining numbers beginning with 1 and ciphers, and such as to bear a certain relation to some prime number by means of which its logarithm may be found. The method is this: Find three products having the common difference 1, and such that two of them are produced from factors having given logarithms, and the third produced

from the prime number, whose logarithm is required, either multiplied by itself, or by some other number whose logarithm is given :
then the greatest and least of these three products being multiplied together, and the mean by itself, there arise two other products also differing by 1, of which the greater, divided by the less, gives for a quotient 1, with a small decimal, having several ciphers at the beginning.
Then the logarithm of this quotient being found as before, from
thence will be deduced the required logarithm of the given prime
number. Thus if it be proposed to find the logarithm of the prime
number 7; here $6 \times 8 = 48$, $7 \times 7 = 49$, and $5 \times 10 = 50$, will be
the three products, of which the logarithms of 48 and 50, the 1st
and 3d, will be given from those of their factors 6, 8, 5, 10 : also
$48 \times 50 = 2400$, and $49 \times 49 = 2401$, are the two new products,
and $2401 \div 2400 = 1,00041\frac{2}{3}$ their quotient: then the least of 44
means between 1 and this quotient is
1,00000,00000,00000,02367,98249,04333,6405, which multiplied by
43429 &c, produces 0,00000,00000,00000,01028,40172,88387,29715,
for its logarithm; which being 44 times doubled, or multiplied by
17592186044416, produces 0,00018,09183,45421,30 for the logarithm of the quotient $1,00041\frac{2}{3}$; which being added to the logarithm
of the divisor 2400, gives the logarithm of the dividend 2401; then
the half of this logarithm is the logarithm of 49 the root of 2401,
and the half of this again gives 0,84509,80400,14256, 82 for the logarithm of 7, which is the root of 49.——The author adds another
example to illustrate this method; and then sets down the requisite
factors, products, and quotients for finding the logarithms of all other
prime numbers up to 100.

The 10th chapter is employed in teaching how to find the logarithms of fractions, namely by subtracting the logarithm of the denominator from that of the numerator, then the logarithm of the
fraction is the remainder : which therefore is either abundant or de-
fective, that is positive or negative, as the fraction is greater or less
than 1.

In the 11th chapter is shown an ingenious contrivance for very accurately finding intermediate numbers to given logarithms, by the
proportional parts. On this occasion, it is remarked, that while the
absolute numbers increase uniformly, the logarithms increase unequally,
with a decreasing increment; for which reason it happens, that either
logarithms or numbers corrected by means of the proportional parts,
will not be quite accurate, the logarithms so found being always too
small, and the absolute numbers so found too great; but yet so however as that they approach much nearer to accuracy towards the
end of the table, where the increments or differences become much
nearer to equality, than in the former parts of the table. And from
this property our author, ever fruitful in happy expedients to obviate
natural difficulties, contrives a device to throw the proportional part,
to be found from the numbers and logarithms, always near the end of
the table in whatever part they may happen naturally to fall. And
it is this : Rejecting the characteristic of any given logarithm, whose

number is proposed to be found, take the arithmetical complement of the decimal part, by subtracting it from 1,000 &c, the logarithm of 10; then find in the table the logarithm next less than this arithmetical complement, together with its absolute number; to this tabular logarithm add the logarithm that was given, and the sum will be a logarithm necessarily falling among those near the end of the table : find then its absolute number, corrected by means of the proportional part, which will not be very inaccurate, as falling near the end of the table: this being divided by the absolute number, before found for the logarithm next less than the arithmetical complement, the quotient will be the required number answering to the given logarithm; which will be much more correct than if it had been found from the proportional part of the difference where it naturally happened to fall: and the reason of this operation is evident from the nature of logarithms. But as this divisor, when taken as the number answering to the logarithm next less than the arithmetical complement, may happen to be a large prime number; it is further remarked, that instead of this number and its logarithm, we may use the next less composite number which has small factors, and *its* logarithm; because the division by those small factors, instead of by the number itself, will be performed by the short and easy way of division in one line. And for the more easy finding proper composite numbers and their factors, our author here subjoins an abacus or list of all such numbers, with their logarithms and component factors, from 1000 to 10000; from which the proper logarithms and factors are immediately obtained by inspection. Thus, for example, to find the root of 10800, or the mean proportional between 1 and 10800 : The logarithm of 10800 is 4,03342,37554,8695, the half of which is 2,01671,18777, 4347 the logarithm of the number sought, the arithmetical complement of which logarithm is 0,98328,81222,5653 ; now the nearest logarithm to this in the abacus is 0,98227,12330,3957, and its annexed number is 9600, the factors of which are 2, 6, 8 ; to this last logarithm adding the logarithm of the number sought, the sum is 0,99898,31107,8304, whose absolute number, corrected by the proportional part, is 99766,12651,6521, which being divided continually by 2, 6, 8, the factors of 96, the last quotient is 103,92304845471; which is pretty correct, the true number being 103,923048454133 $= \sqrt{10800}$.

We now arrive at the 12th and 13th chapters, in which our ingenious author first of all teaches the rules of the Differential Method, in constructing logarithms by interpolation from differences. This is the same method which has since been more largely treated of by later authors, and particularly by the ingenious Mr. Cotes, in his Canontechnia. How Mr. Briggs came by it does not well appear, as he only delivers the rules, without laying down the principles or investigation of them. He divides the method into two cases, namely when the second differences are equal or nearly equal, and when the differences run out to any length whatever. The former of these is treated in the 12th chapter; and he particularly adapts it to the interpolating 9 equidistant means between two given terms, evidently for this reason, that then the powers of 10 become the principal multipliers or divisors, and so the operations performed mentally. The substance of his process is this: Having given two absolute numbers with their logarithms, to find the logarithms of 9 arithmetical means between the given numbers: Between the given logarithms take the 1st difference, as well as between each of them and their next or equidistant greater and less logarithms: and likewise the second differences, or the two differences of these three first differences; then if these second differences be equal, multiply one of them severally by the numbers 45, 35, &c, as in the annexed tablet, dividing each product by 1000, that is cutting off three figures from each; lastly, to $\frac{1}{10}$ of the 1st difference of the given logarithms add severally the first five quotients, and subtract the other five, so

1	45	Additive products.
2	35	
3	25	
4	15	
5	5	
6	5	Subductive products.
7	15	
8	25	
9	35	
10	45	

shall the ten results be the respective first differences to be continually added to compose the required series of logarithms. Now this amounts to the same thing as what is at this day taught in the like case: It is known that if A be any term of an equidistant series of terms, and a, b, c, &c, the first of the 1st, 2d, 3d, &c, order of differences; then the term z, whose distance from A is expressed by x, will be thus, $z = A + xa + x.\frac{x-1}{2}b + x.\frac{x-1}{2}.\frac{x-2}{3}c + $ &c. And if now, with our author, we make the 2d differences equal, then c, d, e, &c, will all vanish, or be equal to 0, and z will become barely

$$= A + xa + x.\frac{x-1}{2}b.$$

Therefore if we take x successively equal to $\frac{0}{10}, \frac{1}{10}, \frac{2}{10}, \frac{3}{10}$, &c, we shall have the annexed series of terms with their differences. Where it is to be observed, that our author had reduced the differences from the 1st to the 2d form, as he thought it easier to multiply by 5 than to divide by 2. Also all the last terms $(x.\frac{x-1}{2}b)$ are set down po-

Series of terms.	The differences.
A	
$A+\frac{1}{10}a+\frac{9}{200}b$	$\frac{1}{10}a+\frac{9}{200}b=\frac{1}{10}a+\frac{45}{1000}b$
$A+\frac{2}{10}a+\frac{16}{200}b$	$\frac{1}{10}a+\frac{7}{200}b=\frac{1}{10}a+\frac{35}{1000}b$
$A+\frac{3}{10}a+\frac{21}{200}b$	$\frac{1}{10}a+\frac{5}{200}b=\frac{1}{10}a+\frac{25}{1000}b$
$A+\frac{4}{10}a+\frac{24}{200}b$	$\frac{1}{10}a+\frac{3}{200}b=\frac{1}{10}a+\frac{15}{1000}b$
$A+\frac{5}{10}a+\frac{25}{200}b$	$\frac{1}{10}a+\frac{1}{200}b=\frac{1}{10}a+\frac{5}{1000}b$
$A+\frac{6}{10}a+\frac{24}{200}b$	$\frac{1}{10}a-\frac{1}{200}b=\frac{1}{10}a-\frac{5}{1000}b$
$A+\frac{7}{10}a+\frac{21}{200}b$	$\frac{1}{10}a-\frac{3}{200}b=\frac{1}{10}a-\frac{15}{1000}b$
$A+\frac{8}{10}a+\frac{16}{200}b$	$\frac{1}{10}a-\frac{5}{200}b=\frac{1}{10}a-\frac{25}{1000}b$
$A+\frac{9}{10}a+\frac{9}{200}b$	$\frac{1}{10}a-\frac{7}{200}b=\frac{1}{10}a-\frac{35}{1000}b$
$A+\quad a$	$\frac{1}{10}a-\frac{9}{200}b=\frac{1}{10}a-\frac{45}{1000}b$

than to divide by 2. Also all the last terms $(x.\frac{x-1}{2}b)$ are set down positive, because in the logarithms b is negative.—If the two 2d differences be only nearly equal, take an arithmetical mean between them, and proceed with it the same as above with one of the equal 2d differences.—He also shows how to find any one single term, independent of the rest; and concludes the chapter with pointing out a method of finding the proportional part more accurately than before.

In the 13th chapter our author remarks, that the best way of filling up the intermediate chiliads of his table, namely, from 20000 to 90000, is by quinquisection, or interposing four equidistant means between two given terms; the method of performing which he thus particularly describes. Of the given terms, or logarithms, and two or three others on each side of them, take the 1st, 2d, 3d, &c, differences, till the last differences come out equal, which suppose to be the 5th differences: divide the first differences by 5, the 2d by 25, the 3d by 125, the 4th by 625, and the 5th by 3125, and call the respective quotients the 1st, 2d, 3d, 4th, 5th *mean* differences; or, instead of dividing by these powers of 5, multiply by their reciprocals $\frac{2}{10}$, $\frac{4}{100}$, $\frac{8}{1000}$, $\frac{16}{10000}$, $\frac{32}{100000}$; that is, multiply by 2, 4, 8, 16, 32, cutting off respectively one, two, three, four, five figures from the end of the products, for the several mean differences: then the 4th and 5th of these mean differences are sufficiently accurate; but the 1st, 2d, and 3d are to be corrected in this manner; from the mean third differences subtract three times the 5th difference, and the remainders are the *correct* 3d differences; from the mean 2d differences subtract double the 4th differences, and the remainders are the correct 2d differences; lastly, from the mean 1st differences take the correct 3d differences, and $\frac{1}{4}$ of the 5th difference, and the remainders will be the correct first differences. Such are the corrections when the differences extend as far as the 5th. However, in completing those chiliads in this way, there will be only 3 orders of differences, as neither the 4th nor 5th will enter the calculation, but will vanish through their smallness: therefore the mean 2d and 3d differences will need no correction, and the mean first differences will be corrected by barely subtracting the 3d from them. These preparatory numbers being thus found, all the 2d differences of the logarithms required, will be generated by adding continually, from the less to the greater, the constant 3d difference; and the series of 1st differences will be found by adding the several 2d differences; and lastly, by adding continually these 1st differences to the 1st given logarithm &c, the required logarithmic terms are generated.

These easy rules being laid down, Mr. Briggs next teaches how by them the remaining chiliads may best be completed: namely, having here the logarithm for all numbers up to 20000, find the logarithm to every 5 beyond this, or of 20005, 20010, 20015, &c, in this manner; to the logarithms of the 5th part of each of these, namely 4001, 4002, 4003, &c, add the constant logarithm of 5, and the sums will be the logarithms of all the terms of the series 20005, 20010, 20015, &c: and these logarithms will have the very same differences as those of the series 4001, 4002, 4003, &c; by means of which therefore interpose 4 equidistant terms by the rules above; and thus the whole canon will be easily completed.

Briggs here extends the rules for correcting the mean differences in quinquisection, as far as the 20th difference; he also lays down similar rules for trisection, and speaks of general rules for any other section, but omitted as being less easy. So that he appears to have been possessed of all that Cotes afterwards delivered in his *Canonotechnia sive Constructio Tabularum per Differentias*, drawn from the *Differential Method*, as their general rules exactly agree, Briggs's mean and correct differences being by Cotes called round and quadrat differences, because he expresses them by the numbers 1, 2, 3, &c, written respectively within a small circle and square.

Briggs also observes, that the same rules equally apply to the construction of equidistant terms of any other kind, such as sines, tangents, secants, the powers of numbers, &c: and further remarks, that of the sines of three equidistant arcs, all the remote differences may be found by the rule of proportion, because the sines and their 2d, 4th, 6th, 8th, &c differences, are continued proportionals, as are also the 1st, 3d, 5th, 7th, &c differences, among themselves; and, like as the 2d, 4th, 6th, &c differences are proportional to the sines of the mean arcs, so also are the 1st, 3d, 5th, &c differences proportional to the cosines of the same arcs. Moreover, with regard to the powers of numbers, he remarks the following curious properties; 1st, that they will each have as many orders of differences as are denoted by the index of the power, the squares having two orders of differences, the cubes three, the 4th powers four, &c; 2d, that the last differences will be all equal, and each equal to the common difference of the sides or roots raised to the given power and multiplied by $1 \times 2 \times 3 \times 4$, &c, continued to as many terms as there are units in the index : so if the roots differ by 1, the second differences of the squares will be each 1×2 or 2, the 3d differences of the cubes each $1 \times 2 \times 3$ or 6, the 4th differences of the 4th powers each $1 \times 2 \times 3 \times 4$ or 24, and so on ; and if the common difference of the roots be any other number n, then the last differences of the squares, cubes, 4th powers, 5th powers, &c, will be respectively $2n^2$, $6n^3$, $24n^4$, $120n^5$, &c.

Besides what was shown in the 11th chapter, concerning the taking out the logarithms of large numbers by means of proportional parts, Briggs employs the next or 14th chapter in teaching how, from the first ten chiliads only, and a small table of one page, here given, to find the number answering to any logarithm, and the logarithm to any number, consisting of fourteen places of figures[*].

Having thus fully shown the construction and chief properties of his logarithms, our ingenious author, in the remaining eighteen chapters, exemplifies their uses in many curious and important subjects; such as the Rule-of-Three, or rule of proportion; finding the roots of given numbers; finding any number of mean proportionals between two given terms; with other arithmetical rules; also various geometrical subjects, as 1st, Having given the sides of any plane-triangle, to find the area, perpendicular, angles, and diameters of the inscribed and circumscribed circles; 2d, In a right-angled triangle, having given any two of these, to find the rest, viz, one leg

---

[*] It is no more than a large exemplification of this method of Briggs's that has been printed so late as 1771, in a 4to tract by Mr. Robert Flower, under the title of *The Radix, A New Way of making Logarithms*. Though Briggs's work might not be known to this writer.

and the hypotenuse, one leg and the sum or difference of the hypotenuse and the other leg, the two legs; one leg and the area, the area and the sum or difference of the legs, the hypotenuse and sum or difference of the legs, the hypotenuse and area, and the perimeter and area; 3d, Upon a given base to describe a triangle equal and isoperimetrical to another triangle given; 4th, To describe the circumference of a circle so, that the three distances from any point in it to the three angles of a given plane triangle, shall be to one another in a given ratio; 5th, Having given the base, the area, and the ratio of the two sides, of a plane triangle, to find the sides; 6th, Given the base, difference of the sides, and area of a triangle, to find the sides; 7th, To find a triangle whose area and perimeter shall be expressed by the same number; 8th, Of four given lines, of which the sum of any three is greater than the fourth, to form a quadrilateral figure about which a circle may be described; 9th, Of the diameter, circumference, and area of a circle, and the surface and solidity of the sphere generated by it, having any one given, to find any of the rest; 10th, Concerning the ellipse, spheroid, and gauging; 11th, To cut a line or a number in extreme and mean ratio; 12th, Given the diameter of a circle, to find the sides and areas of the inscribed and circumscribed regular figures of 3, 4, 5, 6, 8, 10, 12, and 16 sides; 13th, Concerning the regular figures of 7, 9, 15, 24, and 30 sides; 14th, Of isoperimetrical regular figures; 15th, Of equal regular figures; and 16th, Of the sphere and the five regular bodies; which closes this introduction. Such of these problems as can admit of it, are determined by elegant geometrical constructions, and they are all illustrated by accurate arithmetical calculations, performed by logarithms; for the exemplification of which they are purposely given. At the end he remarks, that the chief and most necessary use of logarithms, is in the doctrine of spherical trigonometry, which he here promises to give in a future work, and which was accomplished in his *Trigonometria Britannica;* to the description of which we now proceed.

Of BRIGGS'S *Trigonometria Britannica.*

At the close of the account of writings on the natural sines, tangents, and secants, we omitted the description of this work of our learned author, though it is perhaps the greatest of this kind, all things considered, that ever was executed by one person; purposely reserving my account of it to this place, not only as it is connected with the invention and construction of logarithms, but thinking it deserved more peculiar and distinguished notice, on account of the importance and originality of its contents. The division of the quadrant, and the mode of construction, are both new; and the numbers are far more accurate, and are extended to more places, than they had ever been before. The circular arcs had always been divided in a sexagesimal proportion; but here the quadrant is divided into degrees and decimals, as this is a much easier mode of computation than by 60ths; the division being completed only to 100ths of degrees, though his design was to have extended it to 1000ths of degrees. And, besides his own private opinion, he was induced to adopt this method of decimal divisions, partly at the request of other persons, and partly perhaps from the authority of Vieta, pa. 29 *Calendarii Gregoriani.* And it is probable that computations by this decimal division would have come into general use, had it not been for the publication of Vlacq's tables, which were extended to every 10 seconds, or 6th parts of minutes. But besides this method by a decimal division of the degrees, of which the whole circle contains 360, or the quadrant 90, in the 14th chapter he remarks, that some other persons were inclined rather to adopt a complete decimal division of the whole circle, first into 100 parts, and each of these into 1000 parts; and for *their* sakes he subjoins a small table of the sines of every 40th part of the quadrant, and remarks, that from these few the whole may be made out by continual quinquisections; namely, 5 times these 40 make 200, then 5 times these give 1000, thirdly, 5 times these give 5000, and lastly, 5 times these give 25000 for the whole quadrant, or 100000 for the whole circumference.

But to return. Our author's large table consists of natural sines to 15 places, natural tangents and secants each to 10 places, logarithmic sines to 14 places, and logarithmic tangents to 10 places, each besides the characteristic. A most stupendous performance! The table is preceded by an introduction, divided into two books, the one containing an account of the truly ingenious construction of the table, by the author himself; and the other, its uses in trigonometry, &c, by Henry Gellibrand, professor of astronomy in Gresham College, who remarks in the preface, that the work was composed by the author about the year 1600; though it was only published by the direction of Gellibrand in 1633, it having been printed at Gouda under the care of Vlacq, and by the printer of his *Trigonometria Artificialis*, which came out the same year.

After briefly mentioning the common methods of dividing the quadrant, and constructing the tables of sines, &c, from the ancients down to his own time, he hastens to the description of his own peculiar and truly ingenious method, which is briefly this: having first divided the quadrant into a small number of parts, as 72, he finds the sine of one of those parts, then from it the sines of the double, triple, quadruple, &c; up to the quadrant or 72 parts, He next quinquisects each of these parts; by interposing four equidistant means, by differences; he then quinquisects each of these; and finally, each of these again; which completes the division as far as degrees and centesms. The rules for performing all these things he investigates and illustrates in a very ample manner. In treating of multiple and submultiple arcs, he gives general algebraical expressions for the sine or chord of any multiple whatever of a given arc, which he deduced from a geometrical figure, by finding the law for the series of successive multiple chords or sines, after the manner of Vieta, who was the first person that I know of, who laid down general rules for the chords of multiples and submultiples of arcs and angles : and the same was afterwards improved by Sir I. Newton, to such form, that radius, and double the cosine of the first given angle, are the first and second terms of all the proportions for finding the sines and cosines of the multiple angles. For assigning the coefficients of the terms in the multiple expressions, our author here delivers the construction of figurate or polygonal numbers, inserts a large table of them, and teaches their several uses; one of which is, that every other number, taken in the diagonal lines, furnishes the coefficients of the terms of the general equation by which the sines and chords of multiple arcs are expressed, which he amply illustrates ; and another, that the same diagonal numbers constitute the coefficients of the terms of any power of a binomial; which property was also mentioned by Vieta in his *Angulares Sectiones, theor.* 6, 7 ; and before him, pretty fully treated of by Stifelius, in his Arithmetica Integra, fol. 44 & seq.; where he inserts and makes the like use of such a table of figurate numbers, in extracting the roots of all powers whatever. But it was perhaps known much earlier, as appears by the treatise on figurate numbers by Nichomachus, (see Malcolm's History, p. xviii). Though indeed Cardan seems to ascribe this discovery to Stifelius. See his Opus Novum de Proportionibus Numerorum, where he quotes it, and extracts the table and its use from Stifel's book. Cardan, in p. 135, &c, of the same work, makes use of a like table to find the number of variations, or conjugations as he calls them. Stevinus too makes use of the same coefficients and method of roots as Stifelius. See his Arith. page 25. And even Lucas de Burgo extracts the cube root by the same coefficients, about the year 1470. But he does not go to any higher roots. And this is the first mention I have seen made of this law of the coefficients of the powers of a binomial, commonly called Sir I. Newton's binomial theorem, though it is very evident that Sir Isaac was not the first inventor of it : the part of it properly belonging to him seems to be only the extending it to fractional indices, which was indeed an immediate effect of the general method of denoting all roots like powers with fractional exponents, the theorem being not at all altered. However, it appears that our author Briggs was the first who taught the rule for generating the coefficients of the terms successively one from another, of any power of a binomial, independent of those of any other power. For having shown, in his *Abacus* Παγχρησος (which he so calls on account of its frequent and excellent use, and of which a small specimen is here annexed), that the numbers

Aʙᴀᴄᴜs ΠΑΓΧΡΗΣΤΟΣ.							
H	G	F	E	D	C	B	A
—⑧	—⑦	+⑥	+⑤	—④	—③	+②	①
1	1	1	1	1	1	1	1
9	8	7	6	5	4	3	2
	36	28	21	15	10	6	3
		84	56	35	20	10	4
			126	70	35	15	5
				126	56	21	6
					84	28	7
						36	8
							9

in the diagonal directions, ascending from right to left, are the coefficients of the powers of binomials, the indices being the figures in the first perpendicular column A, which are also the coefficients of the 2d terms of each power (those of the first terms, being 1, are here omitted); and that any one of these diagonal numbers is in proportion to the next higher in the diagonal, as the vertical of the former is to the marginal of the latter, that is, as the uppermost number in the column of the former is to the first or right-hand number in the line of the latter; having shown these things, he thereby teaches the generation of the coefficients of any power, independently of all other powers, by the very same law or rule which we now use in the binomial theorem. Thus, for the 9th power; 9 being the coefficient of the 2d term, and 1 always that of the 1st, to find the 3d coefficient we have $2 : 8 :: 9 : 36$; for the 4th term, $3 : 7 :: 36 : 84$; for the 5th term, $4 : 6 :: 84 : 126$; and so on for the rest. That is to say, the coefficients of the terms in any power m, are inversely as the vertical numbers or first line $1, 2, 3, 4, ...m$, and directly as the ascending numbers $m, m—1, m—2, m—3, ...1$, in the first column A; and that consequently those coefficients are found by the continual multiplication of these fractions $\frac{m}{1}, \frac{m—1}{2}, \frac{m—2}{3}, \frac{m—3}{4}, ...\frac{1}{m}$, which is the very theorem as it stands at this day, and as applied by Newton to roots or fractional exponents, as it had before been used for integral powers. This theorem then being thus plainly taught by Briggs about the year 1600, it is surprising how a man of such general reading as Dr. Wallis was, could be quite ignorant of it, as he plainly appears to be by the 85th chapter of his algebra, where he fully ascribes the invention to Newton, and adds, that he himself had formerly sought for such a rule, but without success: Or how Mr. John Bernouilli, not half a century since, could himself first dispute the invention of this theorem with Newton, and then give the discovery of it to Pascal, who was not born till long after it had been taught by Briggs. *See* Bernouilli's *Works*, vol. 4. *pa.* 173. But I do not wonder that Briggs's remark was unknown to Newton, who owed almost every thing to genius and deep meditation, but very little to reading: and I have no doubt that he made the discovery himself, without any light from Briggs, and that he thought it was new for all powers in general, as it was indeed for roots and quantities with fractional and irrational exponents.

When the above table of the sums of figurate numbers is used by our author in determining the coefficients of the terms of the equation, whose root is the chord of any submultiple of an arc, as when the section is expressed by any uneven number, he remarks, that the powers of that chord or root will be the 1st, 3d, 5th, 7th, &c, in the alternate uneven columns, A, C, E, G, &c, with their signs + or — as marked to the powers, continued till the highest power be equal to the index of the section; and that the coefficients of those powers are the sums of two continuous numbers in the same column with the powers, beginning with 1 at the highest power, and gradually descending one line obliquely to the right at each lower power: so, for a trisection, the numbers are 1 in C, and 1+2 =3 in A; and therefore the terms are —1③ +3① : for a quinquisection, the numbers are 1 in E, 1+4=5 in C, 2+3=5 in A; so that the terms are 1⑤ —5③ +5① : for a septisection, the numbers are 1 in G, 1+6=7 in E, 4+10=14 in C, and 3+4= 7 in A: and so the terms are —1⑦ +7⑤ —14③ +7① : and so on, the sum of all these terms being always equal to the chord of the whole or multiple arc. But when the section is denominated by an even number, the squares of the chords enter the equation, instead of the first powers as before, and the dimensions of all the powers are doubled, the coefficients being found as before, and therefore the powers and numbers will be those in the 2d, 4th, 6th, &c, columns: and the uneven sections may also be expressed the same way: hence, for a bisection the terms will be —1④ +4② : for a trisection 1⑥ —6④ +9② : for the quadrisection —1⑧ +8⑥ —20④ +16② : for the quinquisection 1⑩ —10⑧ +35⑥ —50④ +25② : and so on.

Our author subjoins another table, a small specimen of which is here annexed, in which the first column consists of the uneven numbers 1, 3, 5, &c, the rest being found by addition as before, and the alternate diagonal numbers themselves are the coefficients.

F +⑥	E +⑤	D —④	C —③	B +②	A ①
1	1	1	1	1	1
	7	6	5	4	3
		20	14	9	5
			30	16	7
				25	9
					11

The method is quite different from that of Vieta, who gives another table for the like purpose, a small part of which is here annexed, which is formed by adding, from the number 2, downwards obliquely towards the right: and the coefficients of the terms stand on the horizontal line.

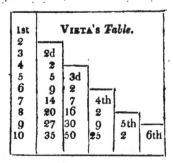

1st	Vieta's *Table.*				
2					
3	2d				
4	2				
5	5	3d			
6	9	2			
7	14	7	4th		
8	20	16	2		
9	27	30	9	5th	
10	35	50	25	2	6th

These angular sections were afterwards further discussed by Oughtred and Wallis. And the same theorems of Vieta and Briggs have been since given in a different form by Herman and the Bernouillis, in the *Leipsic Acts*, and the *Memoirs of the Royal Academy of Sciences.* These theorems they expressed by the alternate terms of the power of a binomial, whose exponent is that of the multiple angle or section. And De Lagny in the same Memoirs, first showed, that the tangents and secants of multiple angles are also expressed by the terms of a binomial, in the form of a fraction, of which some of those terms form the numerator, and others the denominator. Thus, if r express the radius, s the sine, c the cosine, t the tangent, and s the secant, of the angle A; then the sine, cosine, tangent, and secant of n times the angle, are expressed thus, *viz.*

$$\text{Sin.}\,nA = \frac{1}{r^{n-1}} \times \overset{n}{\underset{1}{}}\,\overset{n-1}{\underset{}{}}c\quad s - \frac{n.n-1.n-2}{1.2.3}\,\overset{n-3}{}c\quad s^3 + \frac{n.n-1.n-2.n-3.n-4}{1.2.3.4.5}\,\overset{n-5}{}c\quad s^5\,\&c.$$

$$\text{Cosine}\,nA = \frac{1}{r^{n-1}} \times :c^n - \frac{n.n-1.}{1.2}\,\overset{n-2}{}c\quad s^2 \quad + \frac{n.n-1.n-2.n-3}{1.2.3.4}\,c^{n-4}\,s^4\,\&c.$$

$$\text{Tang.}\,nA = r \times \cfrac{\frac{n}{1}r^{n-1}t - \frac{n.n-1.n-2}{1.2.3.}\,r^{n-3}t^3 + \frac{n.n-1.n-2.n-3.n-4}{1.2.3.4.5}\,r^{n-5}t^5\,\&c.}{r^n - \frac{n.n-1}{1.2.}\,r^{n-2}t^2 + \frac{n.n-1.n-2.n-3}{1.2.3.4.}\,r^{n-4}t^4\,\&c.}$$

$$\text{Sec.}\,nA = r \times \cfrac{s^2\ \text{or}\ r^2+t^2}{r^n - \frac{n.n-1}{1.2}\,r^{n-2}t^2 + \frac{n.n-1.n-2.n-3}{1.2.3.4}\,r^{n-4}t^4\,\&c.}$$

where it is evident, that the series in the sine of nA, consists of the even terms of the power of the binomial $(c\quad s)^n$, and the series in the cosine of the uneven terms of the same power; also the series in the numerator of the tangent, consists of the even terms of the power $(r+t)^n$, and the denominator, both of the tangent and secant, consists of the uneven terms of the same power $(r+t)^n$. And if the diameter, chord, and chord of the supplement, be substituted for the radius, sine, and cosine, in the expressions for the multiple sine and cosine, the result will give the chord and chord of the supplement of n times the arc or angle A. These, and various other expressions, for multiple and submultiple arcs, with other improvements in trigonometry, have also been given by Euler, and other eminent writers on the same subject.

The before mentioned De Lagny offered a project for substituting, instead of the common logarithms, a binary arithmetic, which he called the *natural logarithms*, and which he and Leibnitz seem to have both invented about the same time, independently of each other; but the project came to nothing. De Lagny also published, in several Memoirs of the Royal Academy, a new method of determining the angles of figures, which he called *Goniometry*. It consists in measuring, with a pair of compasses, the arc which subtends the angle in question: yet this arc is not measured by applying its extent to any preconstructed scale, but by examining what part it is of half the circumference of the same circle, in this manner: from the proposed angular point as a centre, with a sufficiently large radius, a semicircle being described, a part of which is the arc intercepted by the sides of the proposed angle, the extent of this arc is taken with a pair of fine compasses, and applied continually upon the arc of the semicircle, by which he finds how often it is contained in the semicircle, with usually a small arc remaining; in the same manner he measures how often this remaining arc is contained in the first arc, and what remains again is applied continually to the first remainder, and so the 3d remainder to the 2d, the 4th to the 3d, and so on till there be no remainder, or else till it become insensibly small. By this process he obtains a series of quotients, or fractional parts, one of another, which being properly reduced into one, give the ratio of the first arc to the semi-circumference, or of the proposed angle, to two right angles or 180 degrees, and consequently that angle in degrees, minutes, &c, if required, and that commonly, he says, to a degree of accuracy far exceeding the calculation of the same by means of any tables of sines, tangents, or secants, notwithstanding the apparent paradox in this expression at first sight. Thus, if the first arc be 4 times contained in the semicircle, the remainder once contained in the first arc, the next 5 times in the second, and finally the fourth 2 times in the third: Here the quotients are 4, 1, 5, 2; consequently the fourth or last arc was $\frac{1}{2}$ the 3d; therefore the 3d was $\dfrac{1}{5\frac{1}{2}}$ or $\frac{2}{11}$ of

the 2d, and the 2d was $\dfrac{1}{1\frac{2}{11}}$ or $\frac{11}{13}$ of the 1st, and the first or arc sought,

was $\dfrac{1}{4\frac{11}{13}}$ or $\frac{13}{63}$ of the semicircle; consequently it contains $37\frac{1}{7}$ degrees,

or $37° \ 8' \ 34''\frac{2}{7}$. Hence it is evident that this method is in fact nothing more than an example of continued fractions, the first instance of which was given by lord Brouncker.

But to return from this long digression; Mr. Briggs next treats of

M

interpolation by differences, and chiefly of quinquisection, after the
manner used in the 13th chapter of his construction of logarithms,
before described. He here proves that curious property of the sines
and their several orders of differences, before mentioned, namely,
that of equidifferent arcs, the sines, with the 2d, 4th, 6th, &c differences, are continued proportionals; as also the cosines of the
means between those arcs, and the 1st, 3d, 5th, &c differences. And
to this treatise, on interpolation by differences, he adds a marginal
note, complaining that this 13th chapter of his *Arithmetica Logarithmica* had been omitted by Vlacq in his edition of it; as if he were
afraid of an intention to deprive him of the honour of the invention of
interpolation by successive differences. The note is this: *Modus
correctionis à me traditus est Arithmeticæ Logarithmicæ capite* 13, *in
editione Londinensi: Istud autem caput unà cum sequenti in editione
Batava me inconsulto et inscio omissum fuit: nec in omnibus, editionis
illius author (vir alioqui industrius et non indoctus), meam mentem
videtur assequutus: Ideoque, ne quicquam desit cuiquam, qui integrum
canonem conficere cupiat, quædam maximè necessaria illinc huc trans-
ferenda censui.*

A large specimen of quinquisection by differences is then given,
and he shows how it is to be applied to the construction of the whole
canon of sines, both for 100th and 1000th parts of degrees; namely,
for centesms, divide the quadrant first into 72 equal parts, and find
their sines by the primary methods; then these quinquisected give
360 parts, a second quinquisection gives 1800 parts, and a third
gives 9000 parts, or centesms of degrees: but for millesms, divide the
quadrant into 144 equal parts; then one quinquisection gives 720, a
second gives 3600, a third 18000, and a fourth gives 90000 parts, or
millesms.

He next proceeds to the natural tangents and secants, which he
directs to be raised in the same manner, by interpolations from a few
primary ones, constructed from the known proportions between sines,
tangents, and secants; excepting that half the tangents and secants
are to be formed by addition and subtraction only, by means of some
such theorems as these, namely, 1st, the secant of an arc is equal to
the sum of the tangent of the same arc, and the tangent of half its
complement, which will find every other secant; 2d, double the tangent of an arc, added to the tangent of half its complement, is equal
to the tangent of the sum of that arc and the said half complement, by
which rule half the tangents will be found; &c.

In the two remaining chapters of this book are treated the construction of the logarithmic sines, tangents, and secants. This is preceded by some remarks on the origin and invention of them. Our
author here observes, that logarithms may be of various kinds; that
others had followed the plan of Baron Napier the first inventor,
among whom Benjamin Ursinus is especially commended, who applied Napier's logarithms to every ten seconds of the quadrant; but
that he himself, encouraged by the noble inventor, devised other lo-

garithms that were much easier and more excellent *. He says he put 10, with ciphers, for the logarithm of radius; 9 for the logarithm sine of 5° 44', whose natural sine is one 10th of the radius; 8 for that of 34', whose natural sine is one 100th of the radius, and so on; thereby making 1 the logarithm of the ratio of 10 to 1, which is the characteristic of his species of logarithms.

To construct the logarithmic sines, he directs first to divide the quadrant into 72 equal parts as before, and to find the logarithms of their natural sines as in the 14th chapter of his *Arithmetica Logarithmica;* after which, this number will be increased by quinquisection, first to 360, then to 1800, and lastly to 9000, or centesms of degrees. But if millesms of degrees be required, divide the quadrant first into 144 equal parts, and then by four quinquisections these will be extended to the following parts, 720, 3600, 18000, and 90000, or millesms of degrees. He remarks, however, that the logarithmic sines of only half the quadrant need be found in this manner, as the other half may be found by mere addition, or subtraction, by means of this theorem, as the sine of half an arc is to half radius, so is the sine of the whole arc to the cosine of the said half arc. This theorem he illustrates with examples, and then adds a table of the logarithmic sines of the primary 72 parts of the quadrant, from which the rest are to be made out by quinquisection.

In the next chapter our author shows the construction of the natural tangents and secants more fully than he had done before, demonstrating and illustrating several curious theorems for the easy finding of them. He then concludes this chapter, and the book, with pointing out the very easy construction of the logarithmic tangents and secants by means of these three theorems:

    1st, As cosine : sine :: radius : tangent,
    2d, As tangent : radius :: radius : cotangent,
    3d, As cosine : radius :: radius : secant.

So that in logarithms, the tangents are found by subtracting the cosines from the sines, adding always 10 or the radius; the cotangents are found by subtracting always the tangents from 20 or double the radius; and the secants are found by subtracting the cosines from 20 the double radius.

The 2d book, by Gellibrand, contains the use of the canon in plane and spherical trigonometry.

Besides Briggs's methods of constructing logarithms, above described, no others were given about that time. For as to the calculations made by Vlacq, his numbers being carried to comparatively but few places of figures, they were performed by the easiest of Briggs's methods, and in the manner which this ingenious man had pointed out in his two volumes. Thus, the 70 chiliads of logarithms,

---

* His words are : " Ego vero ipsius inventoris primi cohortatione adjutus, alios logarithmos applicandos censui, qui multo faciliorem usum habent, præstantiorem. Logarithmus radii circularis vel sinus totius, a me ponitur 10 &c."

from 20000 to 90000, computed by Vlacq, and published in 1628, being extended only to 10 places, yield no more than two orders of mean differences, which are also the correct differences, in quinquisection, and therefore will be made out thus, namely, one-fifth of them by the mere addition of the constant logarithm of 5 ; and the other four-fifths of them by two easy additions of very small numbers, namely, of the 1st and 2d differences, according to the directions given in Briggs's *Arith. Log.* c. 13, p. 31.   And as to Vlacq's logarithmic sines and tangents to every 10 seconds, they were easily computed thus; the sines for half/ the quadrant were found by taking the logarithms to the natural sines in Rheticus's canon ; and then from these the logarithmic sines to the other half quadrant were found by mere addition and subtraction ; and from these all the tangents by one single subtraction.   So that all these operations might easily be performed by one person, as quickly as a printer could set up the types : and thus the computation and printing might both be carried on together.   And hence it appears that there is no reason for admiration at the expedition with which these tables were said to have been brought out.

Of certain Curves related to Logarithms.

About this time the mathematicians of Europe began to consider some curves which have properties analogous to logarithms.   Edmund Gunter, it has been said, first gave the idea of a curve, whose abscisses are in arithmetical progression, while the corresponding ordinates are in geometrical progression, or whose abscisses are the logarithms of their ordinates; but I cannot find it noticed in any part of his writings.   The same curve was afterwards considered by others, and named the *Logarithmic* or *Logistic* curve by Huygens, in his *Dissertatio de Causa Gravitatis,* where he enumerates all the principal properties of this curve, showing its analogy to logarithms.   Many other learned men have also treated of its properties; particularly Le Seur and Jacquier, in their commentary on Newton's Principia; Dr. John Keill, in the elegant little tract on logarithms subjoined to his edition of Euclid's Elements; and Francis Maseres, Esq. Cursitor Baron of the Exchequer, in his ingenious treatise on Trigonometry ; in which books the doctrine of logarithms is copiously and learnedly treated, and their analogy to the logarithmic curve &c fully displayed. —It is indeed rather extraordinary that this curve was not sooner announced to the public; since it results immediately from baron Napier's manner of conceiving the generation of logarithms, by only supposing the lines which represent the natural numbers to be placed at right angles to that on which the logarithms are taken.   This curve greatly facilitates the conception of logarithms to the imagination, and affords an almost intuitive proof of the very important property of their fluxions, or very small increments, to wit, that the fluxion of the number is to the fluxion of the logarithm, as the number is to the subtangent; as also of this property, that, if three numbers be taken very nearly equal, so that their ratios to each other may differ but a little from a ratio of equality, as for example, the three numbers 10000000, 10000001, 10000002, their differences will be very nearly proportional to the logarithms of the ratios of those numbers to each other: all which follows from the logarithmic arcs being very little different from their chords, when they are taken very small. And the constant subtangent of this curve is what was afterwards by Cotes called the *Modulus* of the system of logarithms: and since, by the former of the two properties abovementioned, this subtangent is a 4th proportional to the fluxion of the number, the fluxion of the logarithm, and the number itself; this property afforded occasion to Mr. Baron Maseres to give the following definition of the modulus, which is the same in effect as Cotes's, but more clearly expressed, namely, that it is the limit of the magnitude of a 4th proportional to these three quantities, to wit, the difference of any two natural numbers that are nearly equal to each other, either of the said numbers, and the logarithm or measure of the ratio they have to each other. Or we may define the modulus to be the natural number at that part of the system of logarithms, where the fluxion of the number is equal to the fluxion of the logarithm, or where the numbers and logarithms have equal differences. And hence it follows, that the logarithms of equal numbers or equal ratios, in different systems, are to one another as the *moduli* of those systems. Moreover, the ratio whose measure or logarithm is equal to the modulus, and thence by Cotes called the *ratio modularis*, is by calculation found to be the ratio of 2·718281828459&c to 1, or of 1 to ·367879441171&c; the calculation of which number may be seen at full length in Mr. Baron Maseres's Treatise on the Principles of Life-annuities, pa. 274 and 275.

The hyperbolic curve also afforded another source for developing and illustrating the properties and construction of logarithms. For the hyperbolic areas lying between the curve and one asymptote, when they are bounded by ordinates parallel to the other asymptote, are analogous to the logarithms of their abscisses or parts of the asymptote. And so also are the hyperbolic sectors; any sector bounded by an arc of the hyperbola and two radii, being equal to the quadrilateral space bounded by the same arc, the two ordinates to either asymptote from the extremities of the arc, and the part of the asymptote intercepted between them. And, though Napier's logarithms are commonly said to be the same as hyperbolic logarithms, it is not to be understood that hyperbolas exhibit Napier's logarithms only, but indeed all other possible systems of logarithms whatever. For, like as the right-angled hyperbola, the side of whose square inscribed at the vertex is 1, gives Napier's logarithms; so any other system of logarithms is expressed by the hyperbola whose asymptotes form a certain oblique angle, the side of the rhombus inscribed at the vertex of the hyperbola in this case also being still 1, the same as the side of the square in the right-angled hyperbola. But the areas of the square and rhombus, and consequently the logarithms of any one and the same number or ratio, differing according to the sine of the angle of the asymptotes. And the area of the square or rhombus, or any inscribed parallelogram, is also the same thing as what was by Cotes called the modulus of the system of logarithms; which modulus will therefore be expressed by the numerical measure of the sine of the angle formed by the asymptotes, to the radius 1; as that is the same with the number expressing the area of the said square or rhombus, the side being 1: which is another definition of the modulus, to be added to those we before remarked above, in treating of the logarithmic curve. And the evident reason of this is, that in the beginning of the generation of these areas from the vertex of the hyperbola, the nascent increment of the abscisse drawn into the altitude 1, is to the increment of the area, as radius is to the sine of the angle of the ordinate and abscisse, or of the asymptotes; and at the beginning of the logarithms, the nascent increment of the natural numbers is to the increment of the logarithms, as 1 is to the modulus of the system. Hence we easily discover that the angle formed by the asymptotes of the hyperbola exhibiting Briggs's system of logarithms, will be 25 deg. 44 min. 25¼ sec. this being the angle whose sine is 0·4342944819 &c, the modulus of this system.

Or indeed any one hyperbola will express all possible systems of logarithms whatever, namely, if the square or rhombus inscribed at the vertex, or, which is the same thing, any parallelogram inscribed between the asymptotes and the curve at any other point, be expounded by the modulus of the system; or, which is the same, by expounding the area, intercepted between two ordinates which are to each other in the ratio of 10 to 1, by the logarithm of that ratio in the proposed system.

As to the first remarks on the analogy between logarithms and the hyperbolic spaces; it having been shown by Gregory St. Vincent, in his *Quadratura Circuli & Sectionum Coni*, published at Antwerp in 1647, that if one asymptote be divided into parts in geometrical progression, and from the points of division ordinates be drawn parallel to the other asymptote, they will divide the space between the asymptote and curve into equal portions; hence it was shown by Mersenne, that by taking the continual sums of those parts, there would be obtained areas in arithmetical progression, adapted to abscisses in geometrical progression, and which therefore were analogous to a system of logarithms. And the same analogy was remarked and illustrated soon after by Huygens and many others, who show how to square the hyperbolic spaces by means of the logarithms.

Of Gregory's * Computation of Logarithms.

On the other hand, Mr. James Gregory, in his *Vera Circuli et Hyperbolæ Quadratura*, first printed at Patavi, or Padua, in the year 1667, having approximated to the hyperbolic asymptotic spaces, by means of a series of inscribed and circumscribed polygons, from thence shows how to compute the logarithms, which are analogous to those areas: and thus the quadrature of the hyperbolic spaces became the same thing as the computation of the logarithms. He here also lays down various methods to abridge the computation, with the assistance of some properties of numbers themselves, by which we are enabled to compose the logarithms of all prime numbers under 1000, each by one multiplication, two divisions, and the extraction of the square root. And the same subject is farther pursued in his *Exercitationes Geometricæ*, to be described hereafter.

There are also innumerable other geometrical figures having properties analogous to logarithms: such as the equiangular spiral, the figures of the tangents and secants, &c; which it is not to our purpose to distinguish more particularly.

Of Mercator's † Logarithmotechnia.

In 1668, Nicholas Mercator published his *Logarithmotechnia, sive methodus construendi Logarithmos nova, accurata, & facilis*; in which he delivers a new and ingenious method for computing the logarithms on principles purely arithmetical; which being curious and very accurately performed, I shall here give a rather full and particular account of that little tract, as well as of the small specimen of the quadrature of curves by infinite series, subjoined to it; and more especially as this work gave occasion to the public communication of some of Sir Isaac Newton's earliest pieces, to evince that he had not borrowed them from this publication. So it appears that these two ingenious men had, independent of each other, in some instances fallen upon the same things.

Mercator begins this work with remarking that the word *Logarithm* is composed of the words *ratio* and *number*, being as much as to say the *number of ratios*; which he observes is quite agreeable to the nature of them, for that a logarithm is nothing else but the number of *ratiunculæ* contained in the ratio which any number bears to unity. He then makes a learned and critical dissertation on the nature of

---

* James Gregory was born at Aberdeen in Scotland 1638, where he was educated. He was professor of mathematics in the college of St. Andrews, and afterwards in that of Edinburgh. He died of a fever in December 1675, being only 36 years of age.

† Nicholas Mercator, a learned mathematician, and an ingenious member of the Royal Society, was a native of Holstein in Germany, but spent most of his time in England, where he died in the year 1690, at about 50 years of age. He was the author of many other works in Geometry, Geography, Astronomy, Astrology, &c.

ratios, their magnitude and measure, conveying a clearer idea of the nature of logarithms than had been given by either Napier or Briggs, or any other writer except Kepler, in his work before described; though those other writers seem indeed to have had in their own minds the same ideas on the subject as Kepler and Mercator, but without having expressed them so clearly. Our author indeed pretty closely follows Kepler in his modes of thinking and expression, and after him, in plain and express terms, calls logarithms the measures of ratios; and, in order to the right understanding that definition of them, he explains what he means by the magnitude of a ratio. This he does pretty fully, but not too fully, considering the nicety and subtlety of the subject of ratios; and their magnitude, with their addition to, and subtraction from, each other, which have been misconceived by very learned mathematicians, who have thence been led into considerable mistakes. Witness the oversight of Gregory St. Vincent, which Huygens animadverted on in the Εξετασις Cyclometriæ Gregorii à Sancto Vincentio, and which arose from not understanding, or not adverting to, the nature of ratios, and their proportions one to another. And many other similar mistakes might here be adduced of other eminent writers. From all which we must commend the propriety of our author's attention, in so judiciously discriminating between the mag-

nitude of a ratio, as of a to b, and the fraction $\frac{a}{b}$, or quotient arising

from the division of one term of the ratio by the other; which latter method of consideration is always attended with danger of errors and confusion on the subject; though in the 5th definition of the 6th book of Euclid this quotient is accounted the quantity of the ratio; but this definition is probably not genuine, and therefore very properly omitted by professor Simson in his edition of the Elements. And in those ideas on the subject of logarithms, Kepler and Mercator have been followed by Halley, Cotes, and most of the other eminent writers since that time.

Purely from the above idea of logarithms, namely, as being the measures of ratios, and as expressing the number of *ratiunculæ* contained in any ratio, or into which it may be divided, the number of the like equal *ratiunculæ* contained in some one ratio, as of 10 to 1, being supposed given, our author shows how the logarithm or measure of any other ratio may be found. But this however only by-the-by, as not being the principal method he intends to teach, as his last and best, and which we arrive not at till near the end of the book, as we shall see below. Having shown then that these logarithms, or numbers of small ratios, or measures of ratios, may be all properly represented by numbers, and that of 1, or the ratio of equality, the logarithm or measure being always 0, the logarithm of 10, or the measure of the ratio 10 to 1, is most conveniently represented by 1 with any number of ciphers; he then proceeds to show how the measures of all other ratios may be found from this last supposition. And he explains the principles by the two following examples,

First, to find the logarithm of 100·5*, or to find how many *ratiun-culæ* are contained in the ratio of 100·5 to 1, the number of *ratiunculæ* in the decuple ratio, or ratio of 10 to 1, being 1,0000000.

The given ratio 100·5 to 1, he first divides into its parts, namely, 100·5 to 100, 100 to 10, and 10 to 1; the last two of which being decuples, it follows that the characteristic will be 2, and it only remains to find how many parts of the next decuple belong to the first ratio of 100·5 to 100. Now if each term of this ratio be multiplied by itself, the products will be in the duplicate ratio of the first terms, or this last ratio will contain a double number of parts; and if these be multiplied by the first terms again, the ratio of the last products will contain three times the number of parts; and so on, the number of times of the first parts contained in the ratio of any like powers of the first terms, being always denoted by the exponent of the power. If therefore the first terms, 100·5 and 100, be continually multiplied till the same powers of them have to each other a ratio whose measure is known, as suppose the decuple ratio 10 to 1, whose measure is 1,0000000; then the exponent of that power shows what multiple this measure 1,0000000, of the decuple ratio, is of the required measure of the first ratio 100·5 to 100; and consequently dividing 1,0000000 by that exponent, the quotient is the measure of the ratio 100·5 to 100 sought. The operation for finding this, he sets down as here follows; where the several multiplications are all performed in the contracted way, by inverting the figures of the multiplier, and retaining only the first number of decimals in each product.

* Mercator distinguishes his decimals from integers thus 100ʃ5, or 100|5.

N

	power
100·5000 - -	1
5001 - -	1
1005000	
5025	
1010025 - -	2
5200101 - -	2
1010025	
10100	
20	
5	
1020150 - -	4
0510201 - -	4
1020150	
20403	
102	
51	
1040706 -	8
6070401 -	8
1083068 - -	16
8603801 - -	16
1173035 -	32
5303711 -	32
1376011 -	64
1106731 -	64
1893406 -	128
6043981 -	128
3584985 -	256
5894853 -	256
12852116 -	512

This power being greater than the decuple of the like power of 100, which must always be 1 with ciphers, resume therefore the 256th power, and multiply it, not by itself, but by the next before, viz. by the 128th, thus

3584985 - -	256
6043981 - -	128
6787831 - -	384
1106731 - -	64
9340130 - -	448
5303711 - -	32
10956299 - -	480

This power again exceeding the same power of 100 more than 10 times, I therefore draw the same 448th, not into the 32d, but the next preceding, thus

9340130 - -	448
8603801 -	16
10115994 -	464

This being again too much, instead of the 16th, draw it into the 8th or next preceding, thus

9340130 - -	448
6070401 - -	8
9720329 - -	456
0510201 - -	4
9916193 -	460
5200101 - -	2
10015603 - -	462

Which power again exceeds the limit; therefore draw the 460th into the 1st, thus

9916193 - -	460
5001 - -	1
9965774 - -	461

Since therefore the 462d power of 100·5 is greater, and the 461st power is less, than the decuple of the same power of 100; I find that the ratio of 100·5 to 100 is contained in the decuple more than 461 times, but less than 462 times. Again,

Since the $\begin{Bmatrix}460\\461\\462\end{Bmatrix}$ power is $\begin{Bmatrix}9916193\\9965774\\10015603\end{Bmatrix}$ and the differences $\begin{Bmatrix}49581\\49829\end{Bmatrix}$ nearly equal;

therefore the proportional part which the exact power, or 10000000, exceeds the next less 9965774, will be easily and accurately found by the Golden Rule, thus:

The just power - - - 10000000
and the next less - - - 9965774
the difference - - - 34226; then

As 49829 the dif. between the next less and greater,
: To 34226 the dif. between the next less and just,
:: So is 10000 : to 6868, the decimal parts; and therefore the ratio of 100·5 to 100, is 461·6868 times contained in the decuple or

ratio of 10 to 1. Dividing now 1,0000000, the measure of the decuple ratio, by 461·6868, the quotient 00216597 is the measure of the ratio of 100·5 to 100; which being added to 2 the measure of 100 to 1, the sum 2,00216597 is the measure of the ratio of 100·5 to 1, that is, the log. of 100·5 is 2,00216597.

In the same manner he next investigates the log. of 99·5, and finds it to be 1,99782307. A few observations are then added, calculated to generalise the consideration of ratios, their magnitude, and their affections. It is here remarked, that he considers the magnitude of the ratio between two quantities as the same, whether the antecedent be the greater or the less of the two terms: so, the magnitude of the ratio of 8 to 5, is the same as of 5 to 8; that is, by the magnitude of the ratio of either to the other, is meant the number of *ratiunculæ* between them, which will evidently be the same, whether the greater or less term be the antecedent. And, he further remarks that, of different ratios, when we divide the greater term of each ratio by the less, that ratio is of the greater mass or magnitude, which produces the greater quotient, *et vice versa*; though those quotients are not proportional to the masses or magnitudes of the ratios. But when he considers the ratio of a greater term to a less, or of a less to a greater, that is to say, the ratio of greater or less inequality, as abstracted from the magnitude of the ratio, he distinguishes it by the word *affection*, as much as to say, greater or less affection, something in the manner of positive and negative quantities, or such as are affected with the signs + and —..... The remainder of this work he delivers in several propositions, as follows.

Prop. 1. In subtracting from each other, two quantities of the same affection, to wit, both positive, or both negative; if the remainder be of the same affection with the two given, then is the quantity subtracted the less of the two, or expressed by the less number; but if the contrary, it is the greater.

Prop. 2. In any continued ratios, as $\dfrac{a}{a+b}$, $\dfrac{a+b}{a+2b}$, $\dfrac{a+2b}{a+3b}$, &c. (by which is meant the ratios of a to $a+b$, $a+b$ to $a+2b$, $a+2b$ to $a+3b$, &c.) of equidifferent terms, the antecedent of each ratio being equal to the consequent of the next preceding one, and proceeding from less terms to greater; the measure of each ratio will be expressed by a greater quantity than that of the next following; and the same through all their orders of differences, namely, the 1st, 2d, 3d, &c. differences; but the contrary, when the terms of the ratios decrease from greater to less.

Prop. 3. In any continued ratios of equidifferent terms, if the 1st or least be a, the difference between the 1st and 2d b, and c, d, e, &c. the respective first term of their 2d, 3d, 4th, &c, differences; then shall the several quantities themselves be as in the annexed scheme;

where each term is composed of the first term, together with as many of the differences as it is distant from the first term, and to those differences joining, for coefficients, the numbers in the sloping or oblique lines contained in the annexed table of figurate numbers, in the same manner, he observes, as the same figurate numbers complete the powers raised from a binomial root, as had long before been taught by others. He also remarks, that this rule not only gives any one term, but also the sum of any number of successive terms from the beginning, making the 2d coefficient the first, the 3d the 2d, and so on; thus, the sum of the first 5 terms is $5a + 10b + 10c + 5d + e$.

1st term	- -	a
2d term	- -	$a + b$
3d term	- -	$a + 2b + c$
4th term	- -	$a + 3b + 3c + d$
5th term	- -	$a + 4b + 6c + 4d + e$
&c.		&c.

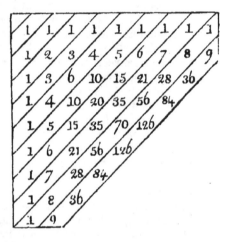

In the 4th *prop.* it is shown, that if the terms decrease, proceeding from the greater to the less, the same theorems hold good, by only changing the sign of every other term, as in the margin.

1st term	- -	a
2d term	- -	$a - b$
3d term	- -	$a - 2b + c$
4th term	- -	$a - 3b + 3c - d$
5th term	- -	$a - 4b + 6c - 4d + e$
&c.		&c.

Prop. 6 and 7 treat of the approximate multiplication and division of ratios, or, which is the same thing, the finding nearly any powers, or any roots of a given fraction, in an easy manner. The theorem for raising any power, when reduced to a simpler form, is this, the m power of $\frac{a}{b}$, or, $(\frac{a}{b})^m$, is $= \frac{s \mp md}{s \pm md}$ nearly, where s is $= a + b$, and $d = a \backsim b$, the sum and difference of the two numbers, and the upper or under signs taking place according as $\frac{a}{b}$ is a proper or an improper fraction, that is, according as a is less or greater than b. And the theorem for extracting the mth root of $\frac{a}{b}$, or $\sqrt[m]{\frac{a}{b}}$, is

$(\frac{a}{b})^{\frac{1}{m}} = \frac{ms \mp d}{ms \pm d}$ nearly; which latter rule is also the same as the former, as will be evident by substituting $\frac{1}{m}$ instead of m in the first theorem. So that universally $(\frac{a}{b})^{\frac{m}{n}}$ is $=\dfrac{ns \mp md}{ns \pm md}$ nearly. These theorems however are nearly true only in some certain cases, namely, when $\dfrac{a}{b}$ and $\dfrac{m}{n}$ do not differ greatly from unity. And in the 7th prop. the author shows how to find nearly the error of the theorems.

In the 8th prop. it is shown, that the measures of ratios of equidifferent terms, are nearly reciprocally as the arithmetical means between the terms of each ratio. So of the ratios $\dfrac{16}{18}, \dfrac{33}{35}, \dfrac{50}{52}$, the mean between the terms of the first ratio is 17, of the 2d 34, of the 3d 51, and the measure of the ratios are nearly as $\dfrac{1}{17}, \dfrac{1}{34}, \dfrac{1}{51}$.

From this property he proceeds, in the 9th prop. to find the measure of any ratio less than $\dfrac{99\cdot5}{100\cdot5}$, which has an equal difference (1) of terms. In the two examples mentioned near the beginning, our author found the logarithm, or measure of the ratio, of $\dfrac{99\cdot5}{100}$, to be $21769\frac{3}{10}$, and that of $\dfrac{100}{100\cdot5}$ to be $21659\frac{7}{10}$; therefore the sum 43429 is the logarithm of $\dfrac{99\cdot5}{100\cdot5}$, or $\dfrac{99\cdot5}{100}, \times \dfrac{100}{100\cdot5}$; or the logarithm of $\dfrac{99\cdot5}{100\cdot5}$ is nearer 43430, as found by other more accurate computations.—— Now to find the logarithm of $\dfrac{100}{101}$, having the same difference of terms (1) with the former; it will be, by prop. 8, as 100·5 (the mean between 101 and 100): 100 (the mean between 99·5 and 100·5) : : 43430 : 43213 the logarithm of $\dfrac{100}{101}$, or the difference between the logarithms of 100 and 101. But the log. of 100 is 2; therefore the logarithm of 101 is 2,0043213.———Again, to find the logarithm of 102, we must first find the logarithm of $\dfrac{101}{102}$; the mean between its terms being 101·5, therefore as 101·5 : 100 : : 43430 : 42788 the logarithm of $\dfrac{101}{102}$, or the difference of the logarithms of 101 and 102. But the logarithm of 101 was found above to be 2,0043213; therefore the logarithm of 102 is 2,0086001.—So that, dividing continually 868596 (the double of 434298 the logarithm of $\dfrac{99\cdot5}{100\cdot5}$ or $\dfrac{199}{201}$) by each number of the series 201, 203, 205, 207, &c, then add 2 to the first quotient, to the sum add the 2d quotient, and so on, adding always the next quotient to the last sum, the several sums will be the respective logarithms of the numbers in this series 101, 102, 103, 104, &c.

The next, or *prop.* 10, shows that, of two pair of continued ratios whose terms have equal differences, the difference of the measures of the first two ratios, is to the difference of the measures of the other two, as the square of the common term in the two latter, is to that in the former, nearly. Thus, in the four ratios

$$\frac{a}{a+b}, \frac{a+b}{a+2b}, \frac{a+3b}{a+4b}, \frac{a+4b}{a+5b};$$ as the measure of $\frac{aa+2ab}{(a+b)}$ (the difference of the first two, or the quotient of the two fractions): is to the measure of $\frac{aa+8ab+15bb}{(a+4b)^2}$ :: so $(a+4b)^2$: is to $(a+b)^2$, nearly.

In *prop.* 11, the author shows, that similar properties take place among two sets of ratios consisting each of 3 or 4, &c, continued numbers.

Prop. 12 shows that, of the powers of numbers in arithmetical progression, the orders of differences which become equal, are the 2d differences in the squares, the 3d differences in the cubes, the 4th differences in the 4th powers, &c. And hence it is shown how to construct all those powers by the continual addition of their differences; as had been long before more fully explained by Briggs.

In the next, or 13th *prop.* our author explains his compendious method of raising the tables of logarithms, showing how to construct the logarithms by addition only, from the properties contained in the 8th, 9th, and 12th propositions. For this purpose, he makes use of the quantity $\frac{a}{b-c}$, which by division he resolves into this infinite series $\frac{a}{b} + \frac{ac}{bb} + \frac{ac^2}{b^3} + \frac{ac^3}{b^4}$ &c (*in infin.*). Putting then $a=100$, the arithmetical mean between the terms of the ratio $\frac{99\cdot5}{100\cdot5}$, $b=100000$, and c successively equal to $0\cdot5$, $1\cdot5$, $2\cdot5$, &c, that so $b-c$ may be respectively equal to $99999\cdot5, 99998\cdot5, 99997\cdot5$, &c, the corresponding means between the terms of the ratios $\frac{99999}{100000}, \frac{99998}{99999}, \frac{99997}{99998}$, &c,

it is evident that $\frac{a}{b-c}$ will be the quotient of the 2d term divided by the 1st, in the proportions mentioned in the 8th and 9th propositions; and when all of these quotients are found, it remains then only to multiply them by the constant 3d term 43429, or rather $43429\cdot8$, of the proportion, to produce the logarithms of the ratios $\frac{99999}{100000}, \frac{99998}{99999}, \frac{99997}{99998}$, &c, till $\frac{10000}{10001}$, then adding these continually to 4, the logarithm of 10000, the least number, or subtracting them from 5, the logarithm of the highest term 100000, there will result the logarithms of all the absolute numbers from 10000 to 100000. Now when $c=0\cdot5$, then

$$\frac{a}{b} = \cdot001, \frac{ac}{bb} = \cdot000000005, \frac{ac^2}{b^3} = \cdot000000000000025, \frac{ac^3}{b^4} = \cdot000000000000000000125,$$

&c.; therefore $\frac{a}{b-c} = \frac{a}{b} + \frac{ac}{bb} + \frac{ac^2}{b^3}$ &c, is $= \cdot001000005000025000125,$

In like manner if $c = 1\cdot5$, then $\frac{a}{b-c}$ will be $= \cdot0010000150002250003375,$

and if $c = 2\cdot5$, then $\frac{a}{b-c}$ will be $= \cdot001000025000625015625,$

&c. But instead of constructing all the values of $\frac{a}{b-c}$ in the usual way of raising the powers, he directs how they may be found by addition only, as in the last proposition. Having thus found all the values of $\frac{a}{b-c}$, the author then shows, that they may be drawn into the constant logarithm 43429 by addition only, by the help of the annexed table of the first 9 products of it.

1	.43429
2	86858
3	130287
4	173716
5	217145
6	260574
7	304003
8	347432
9	390861

The author then distinguishes which of the logarithms it may be proper to find in this way, and which from their component parts. Of these, the logarithms of all even numbers need not be thus computed, being composed from the number 2; which cuts off one-half of the numbers: neither are those numbers to be computed which end in 5, because 5 is one of their factors; these last are $\frac{1}{10}$ of the numbers; and the two together $\frac{1}{2} + \frac{1}{10}$ make $\frac{3}{5}$ of the whole, and of the other $\frac{2}{5}$, the $\frac{1}{3}$ of them, or $\frac{2}{15}$ of the whole, are composed of 3; and hence $\frac{3}{5} + \frac{2}{15}$, or $\frac{11}{15}$ of the numbers, are made up of such as are composed of 2, 3, and 5. As to the other numbers, which may be composed of 7, of 11, &c; he recommends to find *their* logarithms in the general way, the same as if they were incomposites, as it is not worth while to separate them in so easy a mode of calculation. So that of the 90 chiliads of numbers from 10000 to 100000, only 24 chiliads are to be computed. Neither indeed are all of these to be calculated from the foregoing series for $\frac{a}{b-c}$, but only a few of them in that way, and the rest by the proportion in the 8th proposition. Thus, having computed the logarithms of 10003 and 10013, omitting 10023, as being divisible by 3, estimate the logarithms of 10033 and 10043, which are the 30th numbers from 10003 and 10013; and again omitting 10053, a multiple of 3, find the logarithms of 10063 and 10073. Then by prop. 8, say,

As 10048, the arithmetical mean between 10033 and 10063,
to 10018, the arithmetical mean between 10003 and 10033,
so 13006, the difference between the logarithms of 10003 and 10033,
to 12967, the difference between the logarithms of 10033 and 10063.

That is, 1st -- As $\left\{\begin{array}{c}10048 \\ 10078 \\ 10108\end{array}\right\}$: 10018 :: 13006 : $\left\{\begin{array}{c}12967 \\ \&c.\end{array}\right.$

$$\text{Again, As} \begin{Bmatrix} 10058 \\ 10088 \\ 10118 \end{Bmatrix} : 10028 :: 12992 : \begin{Bmatrix} 12953 \\ \&c. \end{Bmatrix}$$

$$\text{And 3dly, As} \begin{Bmatrix} 10068 \\ 10098 \\ \&c. \end{Bmatrix} : 10038 :: 12979 : \begin{Bmatrix} 12940 \\ \&c. \end{Bmatrix}$$

And with this our author concludes his compendium for constructing the tables of logarithms.

He afterwards shows some applications and relations of the doctrine of logarithms to geometrical figures: in order to which, in *prop.* 14, he proves algebraically that, in the right-angled hyperbola, if from the vertex, and from any other point, there be drawn BI, FH perpendicular to the asymptote AH, or parallel to the other asymptote; then will AH : AI :: BI : FH. And,

In *prop.* 15, if AI=BI=1, and HI=a; then will

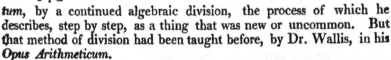

$$FH = \frac{1}{1+a} = 1 - a + a^2 - a^3 + a^4 - a^5 \ \&c, \ in \ infini-$$

tum, by a continued algebraic division, the process of which he describes, step by step, as a thing that was new or uncommon. But that method of division had been taught before, by Dr. Wallis, in his *Opus Arithmeticum.*

Prop. 16 is this: Any given number being supposed to be divided into innumerable small equal parts, it is required to assign the sum of any powers of the continual sums of those innumerable parts. For which purpose he lays down this rule; if the next higher power of the given number, above that power whose sum is sought, be divided by its exponent, the quotient will be the sum of the powers sought. That is, if N be the given number, and a one of its innumerable equal parts, then will

$$a^n + (2a)^n + (3a)^n + (4a)^n \ \&c \dots N^n \ be = \frac{N^n+1}{n-1}:$$ which theorem

he demonstrates by a method of induction. And this, it is evident, is the finding the sum of any powers of an infinite number of arithmeticals, of which the greatest term is a given quantity, and the least indefinitely small. It is also remarkable, that the above expression is similar to the rule for finding the fluent to the given fluxion of a power, as afterwards taught by Sir I. Newton.

Mercator then applies this rule, in *prop.* 17, to the quadrature of the hyperbola. Thus, putting AI=1, conceive the asymptote to be divided from I into innumerable equal parts, namely, Ip=pq=qr =a; then, by the 14th and 15th,

$$\left. \begin{array}{l} ps=1- \ a+ \ a^2- \ a^3 \ \&c \\ qt=1-2a+ \ 4a^2- \ 8a^3 \ \&c \\ ru=1-3a+ \ 9a^2-27a^3 \ \&c \end{array} \right\}$$ But the area BIru is = the sum ps+qt+ru, which is=

$3-6a+14a^2-36a^3$ &c, that is, equal to the number of terms contained in the line Ir, minus the sum of those terms, plus the sum of the squares of the same, minus the sum of their cubes, plus the sum of the 4th powers, &c. Putting now IA = 1, as before, and Ip = 0·1 the number of terms, to find the area BIps: by prop. 16 the sum of the terms will be $\frac{0·1^2}{2}$ = ·005, the sum of their squares = ·000333333, the sum of their cubes ·000025, the sum of the 4th powers ·000002, the sum of the 5th powers ·000000166, the sum of the 6th powers ·000000014, &c. Therefore the area BIps is = ·1 — ·005 + ·000333333 — ·000025 + ·000002 — ·000000166 + ·000000014 &c = ·100335347 — ·005025166 = ·095310181 &c.

Again, putting Iq = ·21 the number of terms, he finds in like manner the area BIqt = ·21 — ·02205 + ·003087 — ·000486202 + ·000081682 — 000014294 + ·000002572 — 000000472 + ·000000088 &c = ·213171345 — ·022550984 = ·190620361 &c.

He then adds, hence it appears that, as the ratio of AI to Ap, or 1 to 1·1, is half or subduplicate of the ratio of AI to Aq, or 1 to 1·21, so the area BIps is here found to be half of the area BIqt. These areas he computes to 44 places of figures, and finds them still in the ratio of 2 to 1.

The foregoing doctrine amounts to this, that if the rectangle BI × Ir, which in this case is expressed by Ir only, be put = *A*, AI being = 1 as before; then the area BIru, or the hyperbolic logarithm of 1 + *A*, or of the ratio of 1 to 1 + *A*, will be equal to the infinite series $A - \frac{1}{2}A^2 + \frac{1}{3}A^3 - \frac{1}{4}A^4 + \frac{1}{5}A^5$ &c; and which therefore may be considered as Mercator's quadrature of the hyperbola, or his general expression of an hyperbolic logarithm in an infinite series.. And this method was further improved by Dr. Wallis in the Philos. Trans. for the year 1668.

In *prop.* 18 Mercator compares the hyperbolic *areolæ* with the *ratiunculæ* of equidifferent numbers, and observes that,
the areola BIps is the measure of the ratiuncula of AI to Ap,
the areola spqt is the measure of the ratiuncula of Ap to Aq,
the areola tqru is the measure of the ratiuncula of Aq to Ar, &c.

Finally, in the 19th *prop.* he shows how the sums of logarithms may be taken, after the manner of the sums of the *areolæ*. And hence infers as a corollary, how the continual product of any given numbers in arithmetical progression may be obtained; for the sum of the logarithms is the logarithm of the continual product. He then remarks, that from the premises it appears, in what manner Mersennus's problem may be resolved, if not geometrically, at least in figures to any number of places. And thus closes this ingenious tract.

In the Philos. Trans. for 1668 are also given some further illustrations of this work, by the author himself. And in various places also in a similar manner are logarithms and hyperbolic areas treated of by Lord Brouncker, Dr. Wallis, Sir I. Newton, and many other learned persons.

Of Gregory's Exercitationes Geometricæ.

In the same year 1668 came out Mr. James Gregory's *Exercitationes Geometricæ,* in which are contained the following pieces:

O

1, Appendicula ad veram circuli et hyperbolæ quadraturam?

2, N. Mercatoris quadratura hyperbolæ geometricè demonstrata:

3, Analogia inter lineam meridianam planisphærii nautici et tangentes artificiales geometricè demonstrata; seu quod secantium naturalium additio efficiat tangentes artificiales: — 4, Item, quot tangentium naturalium additio efficiat secantes artificiales: — 5, Quadratura conchoidis: —— 6, Quadratura cissoidis:—— & 7, Methodus facilis et accurata componendi secantes et tangentes artificiales.

The first of these pieces, or the *Appendicula*, contains some further extension and illustration of his *Vera circuli et hyperbolæ quadratura*, occasioned by the animadversions made on that work by the celebrated mathematician and philosopher Huygens.

In the 2d is demonstrated geometrically, the quadrature of the hyperbola; by which he finds a series similar to Mercator's for the logarithm, or the hyperbolic space beyond the first ordinate (Bl, *fig. pa.* 96.) In like manner he finds another series for the space at an equal distance within that ordinate. These two series having all their terms alike, but all the signs of the one plus, and those of the other alternately plus and minus, by adding the two together, every other term is cancelled, and the double of the rest denotes the sum of both spaces. Gregory then applies these properties to the logarithms; the conclusion from all which may be thus briefly expressed :

since $A - \frac{1}{2}A^2 + \frac{1}{3}A^3 - \frac{1}{4}A^4$ &c $=$ the log. of $\dfrac{1+A}{1}$,

and $A + \frac{1}{2}A^2 + \frac{1}{3}A^3 + \frac{1}{4}A^4$ &c $=$ the log. of $\dfrac{1}{1-A}$,

therefore $2A + \frac{2}{3}A^3 + \frac{2}{5}A^5 + \frac{2}{7}A^7$ &c $=$ the log. of $\dfrac{1+A}{1-A}$,

or of the ratio of $1-A$ to $1+A$.   Which may be accounted Gregory's method of making logarithms.

The remainder of this little volume is chiefly employed about the nautical meridian, and the logarithmic tangents and secants. It does not appear by whom, nor by what accident, was discovered the analogy between a scale of logarithmic tangents and Wright's protraction of the nautical meridian line, which consisted of the sums of the secants. It appears however to have been first published, and introduced into the practice of navigation, by Henry Bond, who mentions this property in an edition of Norwood's Epitome of Navigation, printed about 1645; and he again treats of it more fully in an edition of Gunter's works, printed in 1653, where he teaches, from this property, how to resolve all the cases of Mercator's sailing by the logarithmic tangents, independent of the table of meridional parts. This analogy had only been found to be nearly true by trials, but not demonstrated to be a mathematical property. Such demonstration seems to have been first discovered by Nicholas Mercator, who, desirous of making the most advantage of this and another concealed invention of his in navigation, by a paper in the Philos. Trans. for June 4, 1666, invites the public to enter into a wager with him, on his ability to prove the truth or falsehood of the supposed analogy. But this mercenary proposal it seems was not taken up by any one, and Mercator reserved his demonstration. The proposal however excited the attention of mathematicians to the subject itself, and a demonstration was not long wanting. The first was published about two years after by Gregory, in the tract now under consideration, and from thence and other similar properties, here demonstrated, he shows, in the last article, how the tables of logarithmic tangents and secants may easily be computed, from the natural tangents and secants. The substance of which is as follows:

Let AI be the arc of a quadrant extended in a right line, and let the figure AHI be composed of the natural tangents of every arc from the point A, erected perpendicular to AI at their respective points: let AP, PO, ON, NM, &c, be the very small equal parts into which the quadrant is divided, namely, each $\frac{1}{80}$, or $\frac{1}{100}$ of a degree: draw PB, OC, ND, ME, &c, perpendicular to AI. Then it is manifest, from what had been demonstrated, that the figures ABP, ACO, &c, are the artificial secants of the arcs AP, AO, &c, putting 0 for the artificial radius. It is also manifest, that the rectangles BO, CN, DM, &c, will be found from the multiplication of the small part AP of the quadrant by each natural tangent. But, he proceeds, there is a little more difficulty in measuring the figures ABP, BCX, CDV, &c; for if the first differences of the tangents be equal, AB, BC, CD, &c, will not differ from right lines, and then the figures ABP, BCX, CDV, &c, will be right-angled triangles, and therefore any one, as HQG, will be $= \frac{1}{2}$ QH × QG: but if the second differences be equal, the said figures will be portions of trilineal quadratrices; for example HQG will be a portion of a trilineal quadratrix, whose axis is parallel to QH; and each of the last differences being z, it will be QHG $= \frac{1}{2}$ QH × QG—$\frac{1}{12}$ z × QG: and if the third differences be equal, the said figures will be portions of trilineal cubices, and then shall QHG be $= \frac{1}{2}$ QH × QG—$(\sqrt{} (\frac{1}{12}$ QH × z × QG²—$\frac{1}{1728}$ z² × QG²): when the 4th differences are equal, the said figures are portions of trilineal quadrato-quadratrices, and the 4th differences are equal to 24 times the 4th power of QG divided by the cube of the latus rectum; also when the 5th differences are equal, the said figures are portions of trilineal sursolids, and the 5th differences are equal to 120 times the sursolid of QG divided by the 4th power of the latus rectum; and so on *in infinitum*. What has been here said of the composition of artificial secants from the natural tangents, it is remarked, may in like manner be understood of the composition of artificial tangents, from the natural secants, according to what was before demonstrated. It is also observed that the artificial tangents and secants are computed, as above, on the supposition that 0 is the logarithm of 1, and 1000000000000 the radius, and 2302585092990156240178870 the logarithm of 10; but that they may be more easily computed, namely, by addition only, by putting $\frac{1}{60}$ of a degree $=$ QG $=$ AP $=$ 1, and the logarithm of $10 = 7915704467897819$; for by this means $\frac{1}{2}$QH $\times$ QG is $= \frac{1}{2}$QH $=$ QHG, and $\frac{1}{2}$QH $\times$ QG $- \frac{1}{12}$Z $\times$ QG $= \frac{1}{2}$ QH $- \frac{1}{12}$Z $=$ QHG, also

$$\tfrac{1}{2} QH \times QG - \surd (\tfrac{1}{72} QH \times Z \times QG^2 - \tfrac{1}{1728}Z^2 \times QG^4) = \tfrac{1}{2}QH - \surd (\tfrac{1}{72}QH \times Z - \tfrac{1}{1728}Z^2) = QHG:$$ and finally, by one division only are found the artificial tangents and secants to 1000000000000000, the logarithm of 10, putting still 1 for radius, which are the differences of the artificial tangents and secants, in the table from that artificial radius; and to make the operations easier in multiplying by the number 7915704467897819, or logarithm of 10, a table is set down of its products by the first 9 figures. But if AP or QG be $= \frac{1}{100}$ of a degree, the artificial tangents and secants will answer to 13192340779229703 as the logarithm of 10, the first 9 multiples of which are also placed in the table. But to represent the numbers by the artificial radius, rather than by the logarithm of 10, the author directs to add ciphers, &c.—And so much for Gregory's *Exercitationes Geometricæ.*

The same analogy between the logarithmic tangents and the meridian line, as also other similar properties, were afterwards more elegantly demonstrated by Dr. Halley in the Philos. Trans. for Feb. 1696, and various methods given for computing the same, by examining the nature of the spirals into which the rhumbs are transformed in the stereographical projection of the sphere on the plane of the equator: the doctrine of which was rendered still more easy and elegant by the ingenious Mr. Cotes, in his *Logometria,* first printed in the Philos. Trans. for 1714, and afterwards in the collection of his works published in 1732 by his cousin Dr. Robert Smith, who succeeded him in the Plumian professorship of philosophy in the University of Cambridge.

The learned Dr. Isaac Barrow also, in his *Lectiones Geometricæ, Lect.* XI. *Append.* first published in 1672, delivers a similar property, namely, that the sum of all the secants of any arc is analogous to the logarithm of the ratio of $r + s$ to $r - s$, or radius plus sine to radius minus sine; or, which is the same thing, that the meridional parts answering to any degree of latitude, are as the logarithms of the ratios of the versed sines of the distances from the two poles.

Mr. Gregory's method for making logarithms was further exemplified in numbers, in a small tract on this subject, printed in 1688, by one Euclid Speidell, a simple and illiterate person, and son of John Speidell, before mentioned among the first writers on logarithms.

Gregory also invented many other infinite series, and among them these following, viz. a being an arc, t its tangent, and s the secant, to the radius r; then is

$$a = t - \frac{t^3}{3r^2} + \frac{t^5}{5r^4} - \frac{t^7}{7r^6} + \frac{t^9}{9r^8} \ \&c.$$

$$t = a + \frac{a^3}{3r^2} + \frac{2a^5}{15r^4} + \frac{17a^7}{315r^6} + \frac{62a^9}{2835r^8} \ \&c.$$

$$s = r + \frac{a^2}{2r} + \frac{5a^4}{24r^3} + \frac{61a^6}{720r^5} + \frac{277a^8}{8064r^7} \ \&c.$$

And if τ and σ denote the artificial or logarithmic tangent and secant of the same arc a, the whole quadrant being q, and $e = 2a - q$; then is

$$e = \tau - \frac{\tau^3}{6r^2} + \frac{\tau^5}{24r^4} - \frac{61\tau^7}{5040r^6} + \frac{277\tau^9}{72576r^8} \ \&c.$$

$$\tau = e + \frac{e^3}{6r^2} + \frac{e^5}{24r^4} + \frac{61e^7}{5040r^6} + \frac{277e^9}{72576r^8} \ \&c.$$

$$\sigma = \frac{a^2}{2r} + \frac{a^4}{12r^3} + \frac{a^6}{45r^5} + \frac{17a^8}{2520r^7} + \frac{62a^{10}}{28350r^9} \ \&c.$$

Also if s denote the artificial secant of 45°, and $s + l$ the artificial secant of any arc a, the artificial radius being 0; then is

$$a = \tfrac{1}{2}q + l - \frac{l^2}{r} + \frac{4l^3}{3r^2} - \frac{7l^4}{3r^3} + \frac{14l^5}{3r^4} - \frac{452l^6}{45r^5} \&c.$$

The investigation of all which series may be seen at pa. 298 *et seq.* vol. 1. Dr. Horsley's learned and elegant commentary on Sir I. Newton's works, as they were given in the *Commercium Epistolicum* N° xx, without demonstration, and where the number 2 is also wanting in the denominator of the first term of the series expressing the value of σ.

Such then were the ways in which Mercator and Gregory applied these their very simple series $A - \tfrac{1}{2}A^2 + \tfrac{1}{3}A^3 - \tfrac{1}{4}A^4$ &c, and $A + \tfrac{1}{2}A^2 + \tfrac{1}{3}A^3 + \tfrac{1}{4}A^4$ &c, for the purpose of computing logarithms. But they might, as I apprehend, have applied them to this purpose in a shorter and more direct manner, by computing, by their means, only a few logarithms of small ratios, in which the terms of the series would have decreased by the powers of 10 or some greater number, the numerators of all the terms being unity, and their denominators the powers of 10 or some greater number, and then employing these few logarithms, so computed, to the finding of the logarithms of other and greater ratios, by the easy operations of mere addition and subtraction. This might have been done for the logarithms of the ratios of the first ten numbers, 2, 3, 4, 5, 6, 7, 8, 9, 10, and 11, to 1, in the following manner, communicated by Mr. Baron Maseres.

In the first place, the logarithm of the ratio of 10 to 9, or of 1 to $\frac{9}{10}$, or of 1 to $1 - \frac{1}{10}$, is equal to the series

$$\frac{1}{1 \times 10} + \frac{1}{2 \times 100} + \frac{1}{3 \times 1000} + \frac{1}{4 \times 10000} + \frac{1}{5 \times 100000} \ \&c.$$

In like manner are easily found the logarithms of the ratios of

11 to 10; and then, by the same series, those of 121 to 120, and of 81 to 80, and of 2401 to 2400; in all which cases the series would converge still faster than in the first two cases. We may then proceed by mere addition and subtraction of logarithms, as follows:

$$\text{Log.} \tfrac{11}{9} = \text{L.} \tfrac{11}{10} + \text{L.} \tfrac{10}{9}, \quad \text{L.} \tfrac{110}{10} = \text{L.} \tfrac{2}{1}, \quad \text{L.} \tfrac{80}{16} = \text{L.} \tfrac{81}{16} - \text{L.} \tfrac{81}{80},$$

$$\text{L.} \tfrac{121}{81} = 2\text{L.} \tfrac{11}{9}, \quad \text{L.} \tfrac{9}{4} = 2\text{L.} \tfrac{3}{2}, \quad \text{L.} \tfrac{5}{1} = \text{L.} \tfrac{80}{16},$$

$$\text{L.} \tfrac{121}{80} = \text{L.} \tfrac{121}{11} + \text{L.} \tfrac{81}{80}, \quad \text{L.} \tfrac{12}{4} = \text{L.} \tfrac{10}{9} + \text{L.} \tfrac{9}{4}, \quad \text{L.} \tfrac{5}{2} = \text{L.} \tfrac{10}{4},$$

$$\text{L.} \tfrac{120}{80} = \text{L.} \tfrac{121}{80} - \text{L.} \tfrac{121}{120}, \quad \text{L.} \tfrac{9}{16} = 2\text{L.} \tfrac{3}{4}, \quad \text{L.} \tfrac{2}{1} = \text{L.} \tfrac{5}{1} - \text{L.} \tfrac{5}{2}.$$

Having thus got the logarithm of the ratio of 2 to 1, or, in common language, the logarithm of 2, the logarithms of all kinds of even numbers may be derived from those of the odd numbers, which are their coefficients, with 2 or its powers. We may then proceed as follows:

$$\text{L. } 4 = 2\text{L.} 2, \qquad \text{L. } 100 = 2\text{L. } 10, \qquad \text{L.} 2401 = \text{L.} \tfrac{2401}{2400} + \text{L.} 2400,$$

$$\text{L.} 10 = \text{L.} \tfrac{10}{4} + \text{L.} 4, \quad \text{L. } 8 = 3\text{L.} 2, \qquad \text{L. } 7 = \tfrac{1}{4}\text{L.} 2401,$$

$$\text{L. } 9 = \text{L.} \tfrac{9}{4} + \text{L.} 4, \quad \text{L. } 24 = \text{L.} 8 + \text{L.} 3, \quad \text{L. } 11 = \text{L.} \tfrac{11}{9} + \text{L. } 9,$$

$$\text{L. } 3 = \tfrac{1}{2}\text{L. } 9, \qquad \text{L.} 2400 = \text{L.} 100 + \text{L.} 24, \quad \text{L. } 6 = \text{L. } 2 + \text{L. } 3.$$

Thus we have got the logarithms of 2, 3, 4, 5, 6, 7, 8, 9, 10, and 11. And this is, on the whole, perhaps the best method of computing logarithms that can be taken. There have been indeed some methods discovered by Dr. Halley, and other mathematicians, for computing the logarithms of the ratios of prime numbers to the next adjacent even numbers, which are still shorter than the application of the foregoing series. But those methods are less simple and easy to understand and apply, than these series; and the computation of logarithms by these series, when the terms of them decrease by the powers of 10, or of some greater number, is so very short and easy (as we have seen in the foregoing computations of the logarithms of the ratios of 10 to 9, 11 to 10, 81 to 80, 121 to 120, &c,) that it is not worth while to seek for any shorter methods of computing them. And this method of computing logarithms is very nearly the same with that of Sir Isaac Newton, in his second letter to Mr. Oldenburg, dated October 1676, as will be seen in the following article.

Of Sir Isaac Newton's Methods.

The excellent Sir I. Newton greatly improved the quadrature of the hyperbolical-asymptotic spaces by infinite series, derived from the general quadrature of curves by his method of fluxions; or rather indeed he invented that method himself, and the construction of logarithms derived from it, in the year 1665 or 1666, before the publication of either Mercator's or Gregory's books, as appears by his letter to Mr. Oldenburg, dated Oct. 24, 1676, printed in pa. 634 *et seq.* vol. 3, of Wallis's works, and elsewhere. The quadrature of the hyperbola, thence translated, is to this effect. Let dFD be an hyperbola, whose centre is c, vertex F, and interposed square CAFE = 1. In CA take AB and Ab on each side = $\tfrac{1}{10}$ or 0·1: And, erecting the perpendiculars BD, bd; half the sum of the spaces AD and Ad will be

$$= 0\cdot 1 + \frac{0\cdot 001}{3} + \frac{0\cdot 00001}{5} + \frac{0\cdot 0000001}{7} \quad \&c.$$

and the half diff. $= \frac{0\cdot 01}{2} + \frac{0\cdot 0001}{4} + \frac{0\cdot 000001}{6} + \frac{0\cdot 00000001}{8} \quad \&c.$

Which reduced will stand thus,

1·0000000000000,	0·0050000000000	The sum of these 0·1053605156577 is Ad,
3333333333	250000000	and the differ. 0·0953101798043 is AD,
20000000	1666666	In like manner, putting AB and Ab
142857	12500	each=0·2, there is obtained
1111	100	Ad =0·2231435513142, and
9	1	AD =0.1823215567939.

0·1003353477310. 0·0050251679267

Having thus the hyperbolic logarithms of the four decimal numbers 0·8, 0·9, 1·1, and 1·2; and since $\frac{1\cdot 2}{0\cdot 8} \times \frac{1\cdot 2}{0\cdot 9} = 2$, and 0·8 and 0·9 are less than unity; adding their logarithms to double the logarithm of 1·2, we have 0·6931471805597, the hyperbolic logarithm of 2. To the triple of this adding the logarithm of 0·8, because $\frac{2 \times 2 \times 2}{0\cdot 8} = 10$, we have 2·3025850929933, the logarithm of 10. Hence by one addition are found the logarithms of 9 and 11: And thus the logarithms of all these prime numbers, 2, 3, 5, 11, are prepared. Moreover, by only depressing the numbers above computed, lower in the decimal places, and adding, are obtained the logarithms of the decimals 0·98, 0·99, 1·01, 1·02; as also of these 0·998, 0·999, 1·001, 1·002. And hence, by addition and subtraction, will arise the logarithms of the primes 7, 13, 17, 37, &c. All which logarithms being divided by the above logarithm of 10, give the common logarithms to be inserted in the table.

And again, a few pages farther on, in the same letter, he resumes the construction of the logarithms, thus: Having found, as above, the hyperbolic logarithms of 10, 0·98, 0·99, 1·01, 1·02, which may be effected in an hour or two, dividing the last four logarithms by the logarithm of 10, and adding the index 2, we have the tabular logarithms of 98, 99, 100, 101, 102. Then by interpolating nine means between each of these, will be obtained the logarithms of all numbers between 980 and 1020; and again interpolating 9 means between every two numbers from 980 to 1000, the table will be so far constructed. Then from these will be collected the logarithms of all the primes under 100, together with those of their multiples; all which will require only addition and subtraction; for

$$\sqrt[10]{\frac{9984 \times 1020}{9945}} = 2; \frac{10}{2} = 5; \sqrt{\frac{98}{2}} = 7; \frac{99}{9} = 11; \frac{1001}{7 \times 11} = 13; \frac{102}{6} = 17;$$

$$\frac{988}{4 \times 13} = 19; \frac{9936}{16 \times 27} = 23; \frac{986}{2 \times 17} = 29; \frac{992}{32} = 31; \frac{999}{27} = 37; \frac{984}{24} = 41;$$

$$\frac{989}{23} = 43; \frac{987}{27} = 47; \frac{9911}{11 \times 17} = 53; \frac{9971}{13 \times 13} = 59; \frac{9882}{2 \times 81} = 61; \frac{9849}{3 \times 49} = 67;$$

$$\frac{994}{14} = 71; \frac{9928}{8 \times 17} = 73; \frac{9954}{7 \times 18} = 79; \frac{996}{12} = 83; \frac{9968}{7 \times 16} = 89; \frac{9894}{6 \times 17} = 97.$$

This quadrature of the hyperbola, and its application to the construction of logarithms, are still further explained by our celebrated
author in his treatise on Fluxions, published by Colson in 1736,
where he gives all the three series for the areas AD, Ad, Bd, in general terms, the former the same as that published by Mercator, and
the latter by Gregory; and he explains the manner of deriving the
latter series from the former, namely by uniting together the two series
for the spaces on each side of an ordinate, bounded by other ordinates
at equal distances, every 2d term of each series is cancelled, and
the result is a series converging much quicker than either of the former. And, in this treatise on fluxions, as well as in the letter before
quoted, he recommends this as the most convenient way of raising a
canon of logarithms, computing by the series the hyperbolic spaces
answering to the prime numbers 2, 3, 5, 7, 11, &c, and dividing
them by 2·3025850929940457, which is the area corresponding to
the number 10, or else multiplying them by its reciprocal
0·4329448190392518, for the common logarithms. "Then the
logarithms of all the numbers in the canon which are made by the
multiplication of these, are to be found by the addition of their logarithms, as is usual. And the void places are to be interpolated
afterwards by the help of this theorem : Let n be a number to which
a logarithm is to be adapted, x the difference between that and the
two nearest numbers equally distant on each side, whose logarithms
are already found, and let d be half the difference of the logarithms;
then the required logarithm of the number n will be obtained by add-
ing $d + \dfrac{dx}{2n} + \dfrac{dx^3}{12n^3}$ &c to the logarithm of the less number." This
theorem he demonstrates by the hyperbolic areas, and then proceeds
thus; "The two first terms $d + \dfrac{dx}{2n}$ of this series I think to be accurate enough for the construction of a canon of logarithms, even
though they were to be produced to 14 or 15 figures; provided the
number whose logarithm is to be found be not less than 1000. And
this can give little trouble in the calculation, because x is generally
an unit, or the number 2. Yet it is not necessary to interpolate all
the places by the help of this rule. For the logarithms of numbers
which are produced by the multiplication or division of the number
last found, may be obtained by the numbers whose logarithms were
had before, by the addition or subtraction of their logarithms.
Moreover, by the differences of the logarithms, and by their 2d and
3d differences, if there be occasion, the void places may be more ex-
peditiously supplied; the foregoing rule being to be applied only when
the continuation of some full places is wanted, in order to obtain
those differences, &c." So that Sir I. Newton of himself discovered
all the series for the above quadrature which were found out, and afterwards published, partly by Mercator and partly by Gregory; and
these we may here exhibit in one view all together and that in
a general manner for any hyperbola, namely putting CA$=a$, AF

$= b$, and $AB = Ab = x$; then will $BD = \dfrac{ab}{a+x}$, and $bd = \dfrac{ab}{a+x}$; whence the areas are as below, viz.

$$AD = bx - \frac{bx^2}{2a} + \frac{bx^3}{3a^2} - \frac{bx^4}{4a^3} + \frac{bx^5}{5a^4} \ \&c.$$

$$Ad = bx + \frac{bx^3}{2a} + \frac{bx^3}{3a^2} + \frac{bx^4}{4a^3} + \frac{bx^5}{5a^4} \ \&c.$$

$$Bd = 2bx + \frac{2bx^3}{3a^2} + \frac{2bx^5}{5a^4} + \frac{2bx^7}{7a^6} + \frac{2bx^9}{9a^8} \ \&c.$$

In the same letter also, above quoted, to Mr. Oldenburg, our illustrious author teaches a method of constructing the trigonometrical canon of sines, by an easier method of multiple angles than that before delivered by Briggs for the same purpose, because that in Sir Isaac's way radius or 1 is the first term, and double the sine or cosine of the first given angle is the 2d term of all the proportions by which the several successive multiple sines or cosines are found. The substance of the method is thus: The best foundation for the construction of the tables of sines, is the continual addition of a given angle to itself or to another given angle. As if the angle A be to be added;

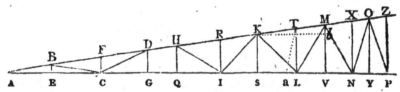

inscribe HI, IK, KL, LM, MN, NO, OP, &c, each equal to the radius AB; and to the opposite sides draw the perpendiculars BE, HQ, IR, KS, LT, MV, NX, OY, &c; so shall the angle A be the common difference of the angles HIQ, IKH, KLI, LMK, &c; their sines HQ, IR, KS, &c; and their cosines IQ, KR, LS, &c. Now let any one of them, LMK, be given, then the rest will be thus found: Draw Ta and Kb perpendicular to sv and MV; now because of the equiangular triangles ABE, TLa, KMb, ALT, AMV, &c, it will be, $AB : AE :: KT : sa \ (= \frac{1}{2}LV + \frac{1}{2}LS)$ $:: LT : Ta \ (= \frac{1}{2}MV + \frac{1}{2}KS,)$ and $AB : BE :: LT : La \ (= \frac{1}{2}LS - \frac{1}{2}LV) :: KT \ (= \frac{1}{2}KM) : \frac{1}{2}Mb \ (= \frac{1}{2}MV - \frac{1}{2}KS.)$ Hence are given the sines and cosines KS, MV, LS, LV. And the method of continuing the progressions is evident. Namely,

as $AB : 2AE ::$
$$\begin{cases} LV : MT + MX :: MX : NV + NY \ \&c \\ MV : NX + LT :: NX : OY + MV \ \&c \end{cases}$$

or $AB : 2BE ::$
$$\begin{cases} LV : NX - LT :: MX : OY - MV \ \&c \\ MV : MT - MX :: NX : NV - NY \ \&c \end{cases}$$

And on the other hand, $AB : 2AE :: LS : KT + KR$, &c.
Therefore put $AB = 1$, and make $BE \times LT = La$, $AB \times KT = sa$, $sa - La = LV$, $2AE \times LV - TM = MX$, &c.

The sense of these general theorems is this, that if P be any one among a series of angles in arithmetical progression, the angle d being their common difference, then as radius or

$$1 : 2 \cos. d :: \begin{cases} \cos. P : \cos. P + d + \cos. P - d \\ \sin. P : \sin. P + d + \sin. P - d \end{cases}$$

$$1 : 2 \sin. d :: \begin{cases} \cos. P : \sin. P + d - \sin. P - d \\ \sin. P : \cos. P + d - \cos. P - d \end{cases}$$

where the 4th terms of these proportions are the sums or differences of the sines or cosines of the two angles next less and greater than any angle P in the series; and therefore subtracting the less extreme from the sum, or adding it to the difference, the result will be the greater extreme, or the next sine or cosine beyond that of the term P. And in the same manner are all the rest to be found. This method, it is evident, is equally applicable whether the common difference d, or angle A, be equal to one term of the series or not: when it *is* one of the terms, then the whole series of sines and cosines becomes thus, viz, as $1 : 2 \cos. d ::$

sin. d : sin. $2d$　:: sin. $2d$: sin. d+sin. $3d$ :: sin. $3d$: sin. $2d$+sin. $4d$ :: sin. $4d$: sin. $3d$+sin. $5d$ &c.
cos. d : 1+cos. $2d$ :: cos. $2d$: cos. d+cos. $3d$ :: cos. $3d$: cos. $2d$+cos. $4d$ :: cos. $4d$: cos. $3d$+cos. $5d$ &c.

which is the very method contained in the directions given by Abraham Sharp, for constructing the canon of sines.

Sir I. Newton remarks, that it only remains to find the sine and cosine of a first angle A, by some other method; and for this purpose, he directs us to make use of some of his own infinite series: thus, by them will be found 1·57079 &c for the quadrantal arc, the square of which is 2·4694 &c; divide this square by the square of the number expressing the ratio of 90 degrees to the angle A, calling the quotient z; then 3 or 4 terms of this series $1 - \dfrac{z}{2} + \dfrac{z^2}{24} - \dfrac{z^3}{720} + \dfrac{z^4}{40320}$ &c, will give the cosine of that angle A. Thus we may first find an angle of 5 degrees, and thence the table may be computed to the series of every 5 degrees, then these interpolated to degrees or half degrees by the same method, and these interpolated again; and so on as far as necessary. But two-thirds of the table being computed in this manner, the remaining third will be found by addition or subtraction only, as is well known.

Various other improvements in logarithms and trigonometry are owing to the same excellent personage; such as the series for expressing the relation between circular arcs and their sines, cosines, versed sines, tangents, &c; namely, the arc being a, the sine s, the versed sine v, cosine c, tangent t, radius 1, then is

$$a = s + \tfrac{1}{6}s^3 + \tfrac{3}{40}s^5 + \tfrac{5}{112}s^7 + \tfrac{35}{1152}s^9 + \tfrac{63}{2816}s^{11} \ \&c.$$

$$a = v^{\frac{1}{2}} + \tfrac{1}{6}v^{\frac{3}{2}} + \tfrac{3}{40}v^{\frac{5}{2}} + \tfrac{5}{112}v^{\frac{7}{2}} + \tfrac{35}{1152}v^{\frac{9}{2}} + \tfrac{63}{2816}v^{\frac{11}{2}} \ \&c.$$

$$a = t - \tfrac{1}{3}t^3 + \tfrac{1}{5}t^5 - \tfrac{1}{7}t^7 + \tfrac{1}{9}t^9 - \tfrac{1}{11}t^{11} \ \&c.$$

$$s = a - \tfrac{1}{6}a^3 + \tfrac{1}{120}a^5 - \tfrac{1}{5040}a^7 + \tfrac{1}{362880}a^9 - \tfrac{1}{39916800}a^{11} \ \&c.$$

$$s = 1 - \tfrac{1}{2}a^2 + \tfrac{1}{24}a^4 - \tfrac{1}{720}a^6 + \tfrac{1}{40320}a^8 - \tfrac{1}{3628800}a^{10} \ \&c.$$

$$v = \tfrac{1}{2}a^2 - \tfrac{1}{24}a^4 + \tfrac{1}{720}a^6 - \tfrac{1}{40320}a^8 + \tfrac{1}{3628800}a^{10} - \tfrac{1}{479001600}a^{12} \ \&c.$$

$$t = a + \tfrac{1}{3}a^3 + \tfrac{2}{15}a^5 + \tfrac{17}{315}a^7 + \tfrac{62}{2835}a^9 + \tfrac{1382}{155925}a^{11} \ \&c.$$

Of Dr. Halley's Method.

Many other improvements in the construction of logarithms are also derived from the same doctrine of fluxions, as we shall show hereafter. In the mean time proceed we to the ingenious method of the learned Dr. Edmund Halley, Secretary to the Royal Society, and the second Astronomer Royal, having succeeded Mr. Flamsteed in that honourable office in the year 1719, at the Royal Observatory at Greenwich, where he died the 14th of January 1742, in the 86th year of his age. His method was first printed in the Philosophical Transactions for the year 1695, and is entitled " A most compendious and facile method for constructing the logarithms, exemplified and demonstrated from the nature of numbers, without any regard to the hyperbola, with a speedy method for finding the number from the given logarithm."

Instead of the more ordinary definition of logarithms, as *numerorum proportionalium æquidifferentes comites,* in this tract our learned author adopts this other, *numeri rationem exponentes,* as being better adapted to the principle on which Logarithms are here constructed, where those quantities are not considered as the logarithms of the numbers, for example, of 2, or of 3, or of 10, but as the logarithms of the ratios of 1 to 2, or 1 to 3, or 1 to 10. In this consideration he first pursues the idea of Kepler and Mercator, remarking that any such ratio is proportional to, and is measured by, the number of equal ratiunculæ contained in each; which ratiunculæ are to be understood as in a continued scale of proportionals, infinite in number, between the two terms of the ratio; which infinite number of mean proportionals is to that infinite number of the like and equal ratiunculæ between any other two terms, as the logarithm of the one ratio is to the logarithm of the other: thus, if there be supposed between 1 and 10 an infinite scale of mean proportionals, whose number is 100000 &c *in infinitum;* then between 1 and 2 there will be 30102 &c of such proportionals; and between 1 and 3 there will be 47712 &c of them; which numbers therefore are the logarithms of the ratios of 1 to 10, 1 to 2, and 1 to 3. But for the sake of *his* mode of constructing logarithms, he changes this idea of *equal* ratiunculæ, for that of other ratiunculæ, so constituted, as that the *same* infinite number of them shall be contained in the ratio of 1 to every other number whatever; and that therefore these latter ratiunculæ will be of *unequal* or different magnitudes in all the different ratios, and in such sort, that in any one ratio, the *magnitude* of each of the ratiunculæ in this latter case, will be as the *number* of them in the former. And therefore if between 1 and any number proposed, there be taken any infinity of mean proportionals, the infinitely small augment or decrement of the first of those means from the first term 1, will be a ratiuncula of the ratio of 1 to the said number; and as the numbers of all the ratiunculæ in these continued proportionals is the same, their sum, or the whole ratio, will be directly proportional to the magnitude of one of the said ratiunculæ in each ratio. But it is also evident that the first of any number of means, between 1 and any number, is always equal to such root of that number, whose index is expressed by the number of those proportionals from 1; so if m denote the number of proportionals from 1, then the first term after 1 will be the mth root of that number. Hence the indefinite root of any number being extracted, the *differentiola* of the said root from unity, shall be as the logarithm of that number. So if there be required the logarithm of the ratio of 1 to $1 + q$; the first term after 1 will be $(1+q)^{\frac{1}{m}}$, and therefore the required logarithm will be as $(1+q)^{\frac{1}{m}}-1$.

But, $(1+q)^{\frac{1}{m}}$ is $=1+\frac{1}{m}q+\frac{1}{m}\cdot\frac{1-m}{2m}q^2+\frac{1}{m}\cdot\frac{1-m}{2m}\cdot\frac{1-2m}{3m}q^3$ &c; or by omitting the 1 in the compound numerators, as infinitely small in respect of the infinite number m, the same series will become

$$1+\frac{1}{m}q+\frac{1}{m}\cdot\frac{-m}{2m}q^2+\frac{1}{m}\cdot\frac{-m}{2m}\cdot\frac{-2m}{3m}q^3 \text{ &c, or by abbreviation it}$$

is $1+\frac{1}{m}q-\frac{1}{2m}q^2+\frac{1}{3m}q^3-\frac{1}{4m}q^4$ &c. and hence, finding the differentiola by subtracting 1, the logarithm of the ratio of 1 to $1+q$

is as $\frac{1}{m}\times(q-\tfrac{1}{2}q^2+\tfrac{1}{3}q^3-\tfrac{1}{4}q^4+\tfrac{1}{5}q^5-\tfrac{1}{6}q^6$ &c.) Now the index m may be taken equal to any infinite number, and thus all the varieties of scales of logarithms may be produced: so if m be taken 1000000 &c, the theorem will give Napier's logarithms; but if m be taken equal to 230258 &c, there will arise Briggs's logarithms.

This theorem being for the increasing ratio of 1 to $1 + q$; if that for the decreasing ratio of 1 to $1 - q$ be also sought, it will be obtained by a proper change of the signs, by which the decrement of the first of the infinite number of proportionals will be found to be $\frac{1}{m}$ into $q+\tfrac{1}{2}q^2+\tfrac{1}{3}q^3+\tfrac{1}{4}q^4$ &c, which therefore is as the logarithm of the ratio of 1 to $1 - q$.

Hence the terms of any ratio being a and b, q becomes $\dfrac{b-a}{a}$, or the difference divided by the less term, when it is an increasing ratio; or $q=\dfrac{b-a}{b}$ when the ratio is decreasing or as b to a. Therefore the logarithm of the same ratio may be doubly expressed; for putting x for the difference $b-a$ of the terms, it will be

$$\text{either } \frac{1}{m} \text{ into } \frac{x}{a}-\frac{x^2}{2a^2}+\frac{x^3}{3a^3}-\frac{x^4}{4a^4} \text{ &c.}$$

$$\text{or } \frac{1}{m} \text{ into } \frac{x}{b}+\frac{x^2}{2b^2}+\frac{x^3}{3b^3}+\frac{x^4}{4b^4} \text{ &c.}$$

But if the ratio of a to b be supposed divided into two parts, namely, into the ratio of a to $\frac{1}{2}a + \frac{1}{2}b$ or $\frac{1}{2}z$, and the ratio of $\frac{1}{2}z$ to b, then will the sum of the logarithms of those two ratios, be the logarithms of the ratio of a to b. Now by substituting in the foregoing series, the logarithms of those two ratios will

$$\text{be } \frac{1}{m} \text{ into } \frac{x}{z} + \frac{x^2}{2z^2} + \frac{x^3}{3z^3} + \frac{x^4}{4z^4} + \frac{x^5}{5z^5} \ \&c.$$

$$\text{and } \frac{1}{m} \text{ into } \frac{x}{z} - \frac{x^2}{2z^2} + \frac{x^3}{3z^3} - \frac{x^4}{4z^4} + \frac{x^5}{5z^5} \ \&c; \text{ and hence the sum,}$$

$$\text{or } \frac{1}{m} \text{ into } \frac{2x}{z} + \frac{2x^3}{3z^3} + \frac{2x^5}{5z^5} + \frac{2x^7}{7z^7} + \frac{2x^9}{9z^9} \ \&c.$$

will be the log. of the ratio of a to b.

Moreover, if from the logarithm of the ratio of a to $\frac{1}{2}z$ be taken that of $\frac{1}{2}z$ to b, we shall have the logarithm of the ratio of ab to $\frac{1}{4}z^2$; and the half of this gives that of $\sqrt{ab}$ to $\frac{1}{2}z$, or of the geometrical mean to the arithmetical mean. And consequently the logarithm of this ratio will be equal to half the difference of that of the above two ratios, and will therefore be $\frac{1}{m}$ into $\frac{x^2}{2z^2} + \frac{x^4}{4z^4} + \frac{x^6}{6z^6} + \frac{x^8}{8z^8}$ &c.

The above series are similar to some that were before given by Newton and Gregory, for the same purpose, deduced from the consideration of the hyperbola. But the rule which is properly our author's own is that which follows, and is derived from the series above given for the logarithm of the sum of two ratios. For the ratio of ab to $\frac{1}{4}z^2$ or $\frac{1}{4}a^2 + \frac{1}{2}ab + \frac{1}{4}b^2$, having the difference of its terms $\frac{1}{4}a^2 - \frac{1}{2}ab + \frac{1}{4}b^2$ or $(\frac{1}{2}b - \frac{1}{2}a)^2$ or $\frac{1}{4}x^2$, which in the case of finding the logarithms of prime numbers is always 1, if we call the sum of the terms $\frac{1}{4}z^2 + ab = y^2$, the logarithm of the ratio of $\sqrt{ab}$ to $\frac{1}{2}a + \frac{1}{2}b$ or $\frac{1}{2}z$ will be found to be

$$\frac{1}{m} \text{ into } \frac{1}{y^2} + \frac{1}{3y^6} + \frac{1}{5y^{10}} + \frac{1}{7y^{14}} + \frac{1}{9y^{18}} \ \&c.$$

And these rules our learned author exemplifies by some cases in numbers, to show the easiest mode of application in practice.

Again, by means of the same binomial theorem he resolves with equal facility the reverse of the problem, namely, from the logarithm given, to find its number or ratio: For, as the logarithm of the ratio of 1 to $1 + q$ was proved to be $(1 + q)^{\frac{1}{m}} - 1$, and that of the ratio of 1 to $1 - q$ to be $\cdots 1 - (1 - q)^{\frac{1}{m}}$; hence, calling the given logarithm L, in the former case it will be $(1 + q)^{\frac{1}{m}} = 1 + L$, and in the latter $(1 - q)^{\frac{1}{m}} = 1 - L$;
and therefore $\left.\begin{array}{l} 1 + q = (1 + L)^m \\ \text{and } 1 - q = (1 - L)^m \end{array}\right\}$, that is, by the binomial theorem,

$$1 + q = 1 + mL + \tfrac{1}{2}m^2 L^2 + \tfrac{1}{6}m^3 L^3 + \tfrac{1}{24}m^4 L^4 + \tfrac{1}{120}m^5 L^5 \ \&c,$$

and $1 - q = 1 - mL + \tfrac{1}{2}m^2 L^2 - \tfrac{1}{6}m^3 L^3 + \tfrac{1}{24}m^4 L^4 - \tfrac{1}{120}m^5 L^5 \ \&c.$

m being any infinite index whatever, differing according to the scale of logarithms, being 1000 &c in Napier's or the hyperbolic logarithms, and 2302585 &c in Briggs's.

If one term of the ratio, of which L is the logarithm, be given, the other term will be easily obtained by the same rule: For if L be Napier's logarithm of the ratio of a the less term, to b the greater, then, according as a or b is given, we shall have,

$$b = a \text{ into } 1 + L + \tfrac{1}{2}L^2 + \tfrac{1}{6}L^3 + \tfrac{1}{24}L^4 \ \&c.$$
$$a = b \text{ into } 1 - L + \tfrac{1}{2}L^2 - \tfrac{1}{6}L^3 + \tfrac{1}{24}L^4 \ \&c.$$

Hence, by help of the logarithms contained in the tables, may easily be found the number to any given logarithm to a great extent. For if the small difference between the given logarithm L, and the nearest tabular logarithm, either greater or less, be called l, and the number answering to the tabular logarithm a, when it is less than the given logarithm, but b when greater; it will follow, that the number answering to the logarithm L, will be

$$\text{either } a \text{ into } 1 + l + \tfrac{1}{2}l^2 + \tfrac{1}{6}l^3 + \tfrac{1}{24}l^4 + \tfrac{1}{120}l^5, \ \&c.$$
$$\text{or } b \text{ into } 1 - l + \tfrac{1}{2}l^2 - \tfrac{1}{6}l^3 + \tfrac{1}{24}l^4 - \tfrac{1}{120}l^5, \ \&c.$$

which series converge so quick, l being always very small, that the first two terms $1 \pm l$ are generally sufficient to find the number to 10 places of figures.

Dr. Halley subjoins also an easy approximation for these series, by which it appears, that the number answering to the log. is nearly

$$\frac{1 + \tfrac{1}{2}l}{1 - \tfrac{1}{2}l} \times a \text{ or } \frac{1 - \tfrac{1}{2}l}{1 + \tfrac{1}{2}l} \times b \left\{ \begin{array}{l} \text{in Napier's} \\ \text{logs. and} \end{array} \right. \frac{n + \tfrac{1}{2}l}{n - \tfrac{1}{2}l} \times a \text{ or } \frac{n - \tfrac{1}{2}l}{n + \tfrac{1}{2}l} \times b \left\{ \begin{array}{l} \text{in Briggs's} \\ \text{logs.;} \end{array} \right.$$

where n is $= 434294481903 \ \&c = \dfrac{1}{m}$.

Of Mr. Sharp's Methods.

The labours of Mr. Abraham Sharp, of Little Horton, near Bradford in Yorkshire, in this branch of mathematics, were very great and meritorious. His merit however consisted rather in the improvement and illustration of the methods of former writers, than in the invention of any new ones of his own. In this way he greatly extended and improved Dr. Halley's method, above described, as also those of Mercator and Wallis; illustrating these improvements by extensive calculations, and by them computing table 5 of this book, consisting of the logarithms of all numbers to 100, and of all prime numbers to 1100, each to 61 places. He also composed a neat compendium of the best methods for computing the natural sines, tangents, and secants, chiefly from the rules before given by Newton; and by Newton's or Gregory's series $a = t - \tfrac{1}{3}t^3 + \tfrac{1}{5}t^5 - \tfrac{1}{7}t^7 \ \&c$, for the arc in terms of the tangent, he computed the circumference of the circle to 72 places, namely from the arc of 30 degrees, whose tangent t is $= \sqrt{\tfrac{1}{3}}$ to the radius 1. Other astonishing instances of his industry and labour appear in his *Geometry Improv'd* printed in 1717, and signed *A. S. Philomath*, from whence the 5th table of logarithms above-mentioned was extracted. This ingenious man was some time assistant at the Royal Observatory to Mr. Flamsteed the first Astronomer Royal; and being one of the most accurate and indefatigable computers that ever existed, he was for many years the common resource for Mr. Flamsteed, Sir Jonas Moore, Dr. Halley, &c, in all intricate and troublesome calculations. He afterwards retired to his native place at Little Horton; where, after a life spent in intense study and calculations, he died the 18th of July 1742, in the 91st year of his age.

Of the Construction of Logarithms by Fluxions.

It appears by the very definition and description given by Napier of his logarithms, as stated in page 42 of this Introduction, that the fluxion of his, or the hyperbolic logarithm, of any number, is a fourth proportional to that number, its logarithm, and unity; or, which is the same, that it is equal to the fluxion of the number divided by the number: For the description shows that $z1 : za$ or $1 :: \dot{z}1$ the fluxion of $z1 : \dot{z}a$, which therefore is $= \dfrac{\dot{z}1}{z1}$; but $\dot{z}a$ is also equal to the fluxion of the logarithm A &c, by the description; therefore the fluxion of the logarithm is equal to $\dfrac{\dot{z}1}{z1}$, the fluxion of the quantity divided by the quantity itself. The same thing appears again at art. 2 of that little piece in the appendix to his *Constructio Logarithmorum*, entitled *Habitudines Logarithmorum & suorum naturalium numerorum invicem*, where he observes that, as any greater quantity is to a less, so is the velocity of the increment or decrement of the logarithms at the place of the less quantity, to that at the greater. Now this velocity of the increment or decrement of the logarithms being the same thing as their fluxions, that proportion is this, $x : a ::$ flux. log. $a :$ flux. log. x; hence if a be $= 1$, as at the beginning of the table of numbers, where the fluxion of the logs. is the index or characteristic c, which is also 1 in Napier's or the hyperbolic logarithms, and 43429 &c in Briggs's the same proportion becomes $x : 1 :: c :$ flux. log. x; but the constant fluxion of the numbers is also 1, and therefore that proportion is also this, $x : \dot{x} :: c : \dfrac{c\dot{x}}{x} =$ the fluxion of the logarithm of x; and in the hyperbolic logarithms, where c is $= 1$, it becomes $\dfrac{\dot{x}}{x} =$ the fluxion of Napier's or the hyperbolic logarithm of x. This same property has also been noticed by many other authors since Napier's time. And the same or a similar property is evidently true in all the systems of logarithms whatever, namely, that the modulus of the system is to any number, as the fluxion of its logarithm is to the fluxion of the number.

Now from this property, by means of the doctrine of fluxions, are derived other ways for making logarithms, which have been illustrated by many writers on this branch, as Craig, John Bernouilli, and almost all the writers on fluxions. And this method chiefly consists in expanding the reciprocal of the given quantity in an infinite series, then multiplying each term by the fluxion of the said quantity, and lastly taking the fluents of the terms; by which there arises an infinite series of terms for the logarithm sought. So, to find the logarithm of any number N; put any compound quantity for N, as suppose $\dfrac{n+x}{n}$

then the flux. of the log. or $\dfrac{\dot{N}}{N}$ being $\dfrac{\dot{x}}{n+x} = \dfrac{\dot{x}}{n} - \dfrac{x\dot{x}}{nn} + \dfrac{x^2\dot{x}}{n^3} - \dfrac{x^3\dot{x}}{n^4}$ &c,

the fluents give log. of N or log. of $\dfrac{n+x}{n} = \dfrac{x}{n} - \dfrac{x^2}{2n^2} + \dfrac{x^3}{3n^3} - \dfrac{x^4}{4n^4}$ &c.

And writing $-x$ for x gives log. $\dfrac{n-x}{n} = -\dfrac{x}{n} - \dfrac{x^2}{2n^2} - \dfrac{x^3}{3n^3} - \dfrac{x^4}{4n^4}$ &c.

Also, because $\dfrac{n}{n\pm x} = 1 \div \dfrac{n\pm x}{n}$, or log. $\dfrac{n}{n\pm x} = 0 - $ log. $\dfrac{n\pm x}{n}$,

theref. log. $\dfrac{n}{n+x} = -\dfrac{x}{n} + \dfrac{x^2}{2n^2} - \dfrac{x^3}{3n^3} + \dfrac{x^4}{4n^4}$ &c.

and log. $\dfrac{n}{n-x} = +\dfrac{x}{n} + \dfrac{x^2}{2n^2} + \dfrac{x^3}{3n^3} + \dfrac{x^4}{4n^4}$ &c.

And by adding and subtracting any of these series, to or from one another, and multiplying or dividing their corresponding numbers, various other series for logarithms may be found, converging much quicker than these do.

In like manner by assuming quantities otherwise compounded for the value of N, various other forms of logarithmic series may be found by the same means.

Of Mr. Cotes's Logometria.

Mr. Roger Cotes was elected the first Plumian professor of astronomy and experimental philosophy in the university of Cambridge, January 1706, which appointment he filled with the greatest credit, till he died the 5th of June 1716, in the prime of life, having not quite completed the 34th year of his age. His early death was a great loss to the mathematical world, as his genius and abilities were of the brightest order, as is manifested by the specimens of his performance given to the public. Among these are his *Logometria*, first printed in number 638 of the Philosophical Transactions, and afterwards in his *Harmonia Mensuarum*, published in 1722 with his other works, by his relation and successor in the Plumian professorship, Dr. Robert Smith. In this piece he first treats in a general way of measures of ratios, which measures, he observes, are quantities of any kind whose magnitudes are analogous to the magnitudes of the ratios, these magnitudes mutually increasing and decreasing together in the same proportion. He remarks, that the ratio of equality has no magnitude, because it produces no change by adding and subtracting; that the ratios of greater and less inequality, are of different affections; and therefore if the measure of the one of these be considered as positive, that of the other will be negative; and the measure of the ratio of equality nothing: That there are endless systems of these, which have all their measures of the same ratios proportional to certain given quantities, called *moduli*, which he defines afterwards, and the ratio of which they are the measures, each in its peculiar system, is called the modular ratio, *ratio modularis*, which ratio is the same in all systems. He then adverts to logarithms, which he considers as the *numerical* measures of ratios, and he describes the method of arranging them in tables, with their uses in multiplication and division, raising of powers and extracting of roots, by means of the corresponding operations of addition and subtraction, multiplication and division.

After this introduction, which is only a slight abridgment of the doctrine long before very amply treated of by others, and particularly by Kepler and Mercator, we arrive at the first proposition, which has justly been censured as obscure and imperfect, seemingly through an affectation of brevity, intricacy, and originality, without sufficient room for a display of this qualification. The reasoning in this proposition, such as it is, seems to be something between that of Kepler and the principles of fluxions, to which the quantities and expressions are nearly allied. However, as it is my duty rather to narrate than explain, I shall here exhibit it exactly as it stands. This proposition is to determine the measure of any ratio, as for instance that of AC to AB, and which is effected in this manner: Conceive the difference BC to be divided into innumerable very small particles, as PQ, and the ratio between AC and AB into as many such very small ratios, as between AQ and AP: then if the magnitude of the ratio between AQ and AP be given, by dividing there will also be given, that of PQ to AP; and therefore, this being given, the magnitude of the ratio between AQ and AP may be expounded by the given quantity $\frac{PQ}{AP}$; for AP remaining constant, conceive the particle PQ to be augmented or diminished in any proportion, and in the same proportion will the magnitude of the ratio between AQ and AP be augmented or diminished: Also, taking any determinate quantity M, the same may be expounded by $M \times \frac{PQ}{AP}$; and therefore the quantity $M \times \frac{PQ}{AP}$ will be the measure of the ratio between AQ and AP. And this measure will have divers magnitudes, and be accommodated to divers systems, ac-

Q

cording to the divers magnitudes of the assumed quantity M, which therefore is called the *modulus* of the system. Now, like as the sum of all the ratios AQ to AP is equal to the proposed ratio AC to AB, so the sum of all the measures $M \times \frac{PQ}{AP}$, found by the known methods, will be equal to the required measure of the said proposed ratio.

The general solution being thus dispatched, from the general expression, Cotes next deduces other forms of the measure, in several corollaries and scholia: as 1st, the terms AP, AQ, approach the nearer to equality as the small difference PQ is less; so that either $M \times \frac{PQ}{AP}$ or $M \times \frac{PQ}{AQ}$ will be the measure of the ratio between AQ and AP, to the modulus M. 2d, That hence the modulus M is to the measure of the ratio between AQ and AP, as either AP or AQ is to their difference PQ. 3d, The ratio between AC and AB being given, the sum of all the $\frac{PQ}{AP}$ will be given; and the sum of all the $M \times \frac{PQ}{AP}$ is as M: therefore the measure of any given ratio, is as the modulus of the system from which it is taken. 4th, Therefore, in every system of measures, the modulus will always be equal to the measure of a certain determinate and immutable ratio; which therefore he calls the modular ratio. 5th, To illustrate the solution by an example: let z be any determinate and permanent quantity, x a variable or indeterminate quantity, and $\dot{x}$ its fluxion; then, to find the measure of the ratio between $z + x$ and $z - x$, put this ratio equal to the ratio between y and 1, expounding the number y by AP, its fluxion $\dot{y}$ by PQ, and 1 by AB: then the fluxion of the required measure of the ratio between y and 1 is $M \times \frac{\dot{y}}{y}$. Now, for y, restore its val. $\frac{z + x}{z - x}$, and for $\dot{y}$ the flux. of that value, $\frac{2z\dot{x}}{(z - x)^2}$, so shall the flux. of the measure become $2M \times \frac{z\dot{z}}{zz - xx}$, or $2M$ into $\frac{\dot{x}}{z} + \frac{\dot{x}x^2}{z^3} + \frac{\dot{x}x^4}{z^5}$ &c.

and therefore that measure will be $2M$ into $\frac{x}{z} + \frac{x^3}{2z^3} + \frac{x^5}{5z^5}$ &c.

In like manner the measure of the ratio between $1 + v$ and 1 will be found to be - - - - M into $v - \frac{1}{2}v^2 + \frac{1}{3}v^3 - \frac{1}{4}v^4$ &c. And hence, to find the number from the logarithm given, he reverts the series in this manner: If the last measure be called m, we shall have $\frac{m}{M}$ or $Q = v - \frac{1}{2}v^2 + \frac{1}{3}v^3 - \frac{1}{4}v^4 + \frac{1}{5}v^5$ &c,

$$\text{therefore } Q^2 = \quad - \quad v^2 - v^3 + \tfrac{11}{12}v^4 - \tfrac{5}{8}v^5 \text{ &c,}$$
$$\text{and } Q^3 = \quad - \quad - \quad - \quad v^3 - \tfrac{3}{2}v^4 + \tfrac{7}{4}v^5 \text{ &c,}$$
$$\text{and } Q^4 = \quad - \quad - \quad - \quad - \quad - \quad v^4 - 2v^5 \text{ &c,}$$
$$\text{and } Q^5 = \quad - \quad - \quad - \quad - \quad - \quad - \quad - \quad v^5 \text{ &c;}$$

then, by adding continually, we shall have,

$$Q + \tfrac{1}{2}Q^2 = v - \tfrac{1}{6}v^3 + \tfrac{5}{24}v^4 - \tfrac{13}{60}v^5 \ \&c,$$
$$Q + \tfrac{1}{2}Q^2 + \tfrac{1}{6}Q^3 = v - \tfrac{1}{24}v^4 + \tfrac{1}{40}v^5 \ \&c,$$
$$Q + \tfrac{1}{2}Q^2 + \tfrac{1}{6}Q^3 + \tfrac{1}{24}Q^4 = v - \tfrac{1}{120}v^5 \ \&c,$$
$$Q + \tfrac{1}{2}Q^2 + \tfrac{1}{6}Q^3 + \tfrac{1}{24}Q^4 + \tfrac{1}{120}Q^5 = v \ \&c,$$

that is $v = Q + \tfrac{1}{2}Q^2 + \tfrac{1}{6}Q^3 + \tfrac{1}{24}Q^4 + \tfrac{1}{120}Q^5 \ \&c$. And therefore the required ratio of $1 + v$ to 1, is equal to the ratio of $1 + Q + \tfrac{1}{2}Q^2$ &c to 1. Put now $m = M$, or $Q = 1$, and the above will become the ratio of $1 + \tfrac{1}{1} + \tfrac{1}{2} + \tfrac{1}{6} + \tfrac{1}{24} + \tfrac{1}{120}$ &c to 1, for the constant modular ratio. In like manner, if the ratio between 1 and $1 - v$ be proposed, the measure of this ratio will come out M into

$$v + \tfrac{1}{2}v^2 + \tfrac{1}{3}v^3 + \tfrac{1}{4}v^4 \ \&c;$$ which being called m, and $\dfrac{m}{M} = Q$,

that ratio will be the ratio of 1 to $1 - Q + \tfrac{1}{2}Q^2 - \tfrac{1}{6}Q^3 + \tfrac{1}{24}Q^4$ &c. And hence, taking $m = M$, or $Q = 1$, the said modular ratio will also be the ratio of 1 to $1 - \tfrac{1}{1} + \tfrac{1}{2} - \tfrac{1}{6} + \tfrac{1}{24} - \tfrac{1}{120}$ &c. And the former of these expressions, for the modular ratio, comes out the ratio of 2,718281828459 &c to 1, and the latter the ratio of 1 to 0,367879441171 &c, which number is the reciprocal of the former.

In the 2d prop. the learned author gives directions for constructing Briggs's canon of logarithms, namely, first by the general series $2 M$ into $\dfrac{x}{z} + \dfrac{x^3}{3z^3} + \dfrac{x^5}{5z^5}$ &c, finding the logarithms of a few such ratios as that of 126 to 125, 225 to 224, 2401 to 2400, 4375 to 4374, &c, from whence the logarithm of 10 will be found to be 2,302585092994 &c, when M is 1; but since Briggs's log. of 10 is 1, therefore as 2,302585 &c is to the modulus 1, so is 1 (Briggs's log. of 10) to 0,434294481903 &c, which therefore is the modulus of Briggs's logarithms. Hence he deduces the logarithms of 7, 5, 3, and 2. In like manner are the logarithms of other prime numbers to be found, and from them the logarithms of composite numbers by addition and subtraction only.

Cotes then remarks, that the first term of the general series $2 M$ into $\dfrac{x}{z} + \dfrac{x^3}{3z^3} + \dfrac{x^5}{5z^5}$ &c, will be sufficient for the logarithms of intermediate numbers between those in the table, or even for numbers beyond the limits of the table. Thus, to find the logarithm answering to an intermediate number; let a and e be two numbers, the one the given number, and the other the nearest tabular number, a being the greater, and e the less of them; put $z = a + e$ their sum, $x = a - e$ their difference, $\lambda =$ the logarithm of the ratio of a to e, that is the excess of the logarithm of a above that of e: so shall the said difference of their logarithms be $\lambda = 2 M \times \dfrac{x}{z}$ very nearly.

And, if there be required the number answering to any given intermediate logarithm, because λ is $=$

$$\dfrac{2Mx}{z} = \dfrac{2Mx}{2a-} \ \text{or} \ \dfrac{2Mx}{2e+x}, \ \text{therefore} \ x = \dfrac{\lambda a}{M + \tfrac{1}{2}\lambda} \ \text{or} \ \dfrac{\lambda e}{M - \tfrac{1}{2}\lambda} \ \text{very nearly.}$$

In the 3d prop. the ingenious author teaches how to convert the canon of logarithms into logarithms of any other system, by means of their *moduli*. And, in several more propositions, he exemplifies the canon of logarithms in the solution of various important problems in geometry and physics; such as the quadrature of the hyperbola, the description of the logistica, the equi-angular spiral, the nautical meridian, &c; the descent of bodies in resisting mediums, the density of the atmosphere at any altitude, &c, &c.

Of Dr. Taylor's Construction of Logarithms.

Dr. Brook Taylor (a very learned mathematician, and secretary to the Royal Society, who died at Somerset-house, Nov. 1731) gave the following method of constructing logarithms, in number 352 of the Philosophical Transactions. His. method is founded on these three considerations : 1st, that the sum of the logarithms of any two numbers is the logarithm of the product of those numbers; 2d, that the logarithm of 1 is nothing, and consequently that the nearer any number is to 1, the nearer will its logarithm be to 0; 3d, that the product of two numbers or factors, of which the one is greater, and the other less than 1, is nearer to 1 than that factor is which is on the same side of 1 with itself; so of the two numbers $\frac{2}{3}$ and $\frac{4}{5}$, the product $\frac{8}{9}$ is less than 1, but yet nearer to it than $\frac{4}{5}$ is, which is also less than 1. On these principles he founds the present approximation, which he explains by the following example. To find the relation between the logarithms of 2 and 10 : In order to this, he assumes two fractions, as $\dfrac{128}{100}$ and $\dfrac{8}{10}$, or $\dfrac{2^7}{10^2}$ and $\dfrac{2^3}{10}$, whose numerators are powers of 2, and their denominators powers of 10, the one fraction being greater and the other less than unity or 1. Having set these two down, in the form of decimal fractions, below each other, in the first column of the following table, and in the second column A and B for their logarithms, expressing by an equation how

1,280000000000	A = . . =	7l2 —	2l10	l2 ⊐ 0,28
0,800000000000	B = . . =	3l2 —	l10	∠0,33
1,024000000000	C = A + B =	10l2 —	3l10	⊐0,300
0,990352031749	D = B + 9c =	93l2 —	28l10	∠0,30107
1,004336277664	E = c + 2D =	169l2 —	59l10	⊐0,301020
0,998959536107	F = D + 2E =	485l2 —	146l10	∠0,3010309
1,000162394165	G = E + 4F =	2136l2 —	643l10	⊐0,30102996
0,999936281874	H = F + 6G =	13301l2 —	4004l10	∠0,301029997
1,000035441215	I = G + 2H =	28738l2 —	8651l10	⊐0,3010299951
0,999971720830	K = H + I =	42039l2 —	12655l10	∠0,3010299959
1,000007161046	L = I + K =	70777l2 —	21306l10	⊐0,30102999562
0,999993203514	M = K + 3L =	254370l2 —	76573l10	∠0,30102999567
1,000000364511	N = L + M =	325147l2 —	97879l10	⊐0,3010299956635
0,999999764687	O = M + 18 N =	6107016l2 —	1838335l10	∠0,3010299956640
comp. ar. 235313				
0=364511O	+ 235313N = 230258582516 7l2 — 693147400972l10			⊐0,3010299956663987

they are composed of the logarithms of 2 and 10, the numbers in question, those logarithms being denoted thus, $l2$ and $l10$. Then multiplying the two numbers in the first column together, there is produced a third number 1,024, against which is written c, for its logarithm, expressing likewise by an equation in what manner c is formed of the foregoing logarithms A and B. And in the same manner the calculation is continued throughout; only observing this compendium, that before multiplying the two last numbers already entered in the table, to consider what power of one of them must be used to bring the product the nearest that can be to unity. Now after having continued the table a little way, this is found by only dividing the differences of the numbers from unity one by the other, and taking the nearest quotient for the index of the power sought. Thus the second and third numbers in the table being 0,8 and 1,024, their differences from unity are 0,200 and 0,024; hence $0,200 \div 0,024$ gives 9 for the index; and therefore multiplying the 9th power of 1,024 by 0,8 produces the next number 0,990352031429, whose logarithm is $D = B + 9c$.

When the calculation is continued in this manner till the numbers become small enough, or near enough to 1, the last logarithm is supposed equal to nothing, which gives an equation expressing the relation of the logarithms, and from thence the required logarithm is determined. Thus, supposing $G = 0$, we have $2136 l2 - 643 l10 = 0$, and hence, because the logarithm of 10 is 1, we obtain $l2 = \dfrac{643}{2136} = 0,30102996$, too small in the last figure only; which so happens, because the number corresponding to G is greater than 1. And in this manner are all the numbers in the third or last column obtained, which are continual approximations to the logarithm of 2.

There is another expedient, which renders this calculation still shorter, and it is founded on this consideration: that when x is small, $(1+x)^n$ is nearly $= 1 + nx$. Hence if $1+x$ and $1-z$ be the two last numbers already found in the first column of the table, the product of their powers $(1+x)^m \times (1-z)^n$ will be nearly $= 1$; and hence the relation of m and n may be thus found, $(1+x)^m \times (1-z)^n$ is nearly $= (1+mx) \times (1-nz) = 1 + mx - nz - mnxz = 1 + mx - nz$ nearly, which being also $= 1$ nearly, therefore $m : n :: z : x :: l.(1-z) : l.(1+x)$; whence $xl.(1-z) + zl.(1+x) = 0$. For example, let 1,024 and 0,990352 be the last numbers in the table, their logarithms being c and D: here we have $1,024 = 1 + x$, and $0,990352 = 1 - z$; consequently, $x = 0,024$, and $z = 0,009648$, and hence the ratio $\dfrac{z}{x}$ in small numbers is $\dfrac{201}{500}$. So that, for finding the logarithms proposed, we may take $500 D + 201 c = 4851 l2 - 14603 l10$

$=0$; which gives $l2=0{,}3010307$. And in this manner are found the numbers in the last line of the table.

Of Mr. Long's Method.

In number 339 of the Philosophical Transactions, are given a brief table and method for finding the logarithm to any number, and the number to any logarithm, by Mr. John Long, B.D. Fellow of C. C. C. Oxon. This table and method are similar to those described in chap. 14, of Briggs's *Arith. Logar.* differing only in this, that in this table, by Mr. Long, the logarithms, in each class, are in arithmetical progression, the common difference being 1; but in Briggs's little table, the column of natural numbers has the like common difference. The table consists of eight classes of logarithms, and their corresponding numbers, as follow:

Lo.	Nat. Numb.	Log.	Nat. Numb.	Log.	Nat. Numb.	Log.	Nat. Numb.
,9	7,943282347	,009	1,020939484	,00009	1,000207254	,0000009	1,000002072
,8	6,309573445	8	1,018591388	8	1,000184224	8	1,000001842
,7	5,011872336	7	1,016248694	7	1,000161194	7	1,000001611
,6	3,981071706	6	1,013911386	6	1,000138165	6	1,000001381
,5	3,162277660	5	1,011579454	5	1,000115136	5	1,000001151
,4	2,511886432	4	1,009252886	4	1,000092106	4	1,000000921
,3	1,995262315	3	1,006931669	3	1,000069080	3	1,000000690
,2	1,584893193	2	1,004615794	2	1,000046053	2	1,000000460
,1	1,258925412	1	1,002305238	1	1,000023026	1	1,000000230
,09	1,230268771	,0009	1,002074475	,000009	1,000020724	,00000009	1,000000207
8	1,202264435	8	1,001843766	8	1,000018421	8	1,000000184
7	1,174897555	7	1,001613109	7	1,000016118	7	1,000000161
6	1,148153621	6	1,001382506	6	1,000013816	6	1,000000138
5	1,122018454	5	1,001151956	5	1,000011513	5	1,000000115
4	1,096478196	4	1,000921459	4	1,000009210	4	1,000000092
3	1,071519305	3	1,000691015	3	1,000006908	3	1,000000069
2	1,047128548	2	1,000460623	2	1,000004605	2	1,000000046
1	1,023292992	1	1,000230285	1	1,000002302	1	1,000000023

where, because the logarithms in each class are the continual multiples 1, 2, 3, &c. of the lowest, it is evident that the natural numbers are so many scales of geometrical proportionals, the lowest being the common ratio, or the ascending numbers are the 1, 2, 3, &c, powers of the lowest, as expressed by the figures 1, 2, 3, &c, of their corresponding logarithms. Also the last number in the first, second, third, &c, class, is the 10th, 100th, 1000th, &c, root of 10; and any number in any class is the 10th power of the corresponding number in the next following class.

To find the logarithm of any number, as suppose of 2000, by this table, look in the first class for the number next less than the first figure 2, and it is 1,995262315, against which is 3 for the first figure of the logarithm sought. Again, dividing 2, the number proposed, by 1,995262315, the number found in the table, the quotient is 1,002374467; which being looked for in the second class of the table, and finding neither its equal nor a less, 0 is therefore to be taken for the second figure of the logarithm; and the same quotient 1,002374467 being looked for in the third class, the next less is there found to be 1,002305238, against which is 1 for the third figure of the logarithm; and dividing the quotient 1,002374467 by the said next less number 1,002305238, the new quotient is 1,000069070; which being sought in the fourth class gives 0, but sought in the fifth class gives 2, which are the fourth and fifth figures of the logarithm sought: again, dividing the last quotient by 1,000046053, the next less number in the table, the quotient is 1,000023015, which gives 9 in the 6th class for the 6th figure of the logarithm sought: and again dividing the last quotient by 1,000020724, the next less number, the quotient is 1,000002291, the next less than which, in the 7th class, gives 9 for the 7th figure of the logarithm: and dividing the last quotient by 1,000002072, the quotient is 1,000000219, which gives 9 in the 8th class for the 8th figure of the logarithm: and again the last quotient 1,000000219, being divided by 1,000000207, the next less, the quotient 1,000000012 gives 5 in the same 8th class, when one figure is cut off, for the 9th figure of the logarithm sought. All which figures collected together give 3,301029995 for Briggs's logarithm of 2000, the index 3 being supplied; which logarithm is true in the last figure.

To find the number answering to any given logarithm, as suppose to 3,30101300: omitting the characteristic, against the other figures 3, 0, 1, 0, 3, 0, 0, as in the first column in the margin, are the several numbers as in the 2d column, found from their respective 1st, 2d, 3d, &c classes; the effective numbers of which multiplied continually together, the last product is 2,000000019966, which, because the characteristic is 3, gives 2000,000019966, or 2000 only, for the required number, answering to the given logarithm.

3	1,995262315
0	0
1	1,002305238
0	0
3	1,000069080
0	0
0	0

Of Mr. Jones's Method.

In the 61st volume of the Philosophical Transactions, is a small paper on logarithms, which had been drawn up, and left unpublished by the learned and ingenious William Jones, Esq. The method contained in this memoir, depends on an application of the doctrine of fluxions, to some properties drawn from the nature of the exponents of powers. Here all numbers are considered as some certain powers of a constant determinate root: so, any number x may be considered as the z power of any root r, or, that $x = r^z$ is a general expression for all numbers, in terms of the constant root r, and a variable exponent z. Now the index z being the logarithm of the number x, therefore, to find this logarithm, is the same thing, as to find what power of the radical r is equal to the number x.

From this principle, the relation between the fluxions of any number, x, and its logarithm z, is thus determined; Put $r = 1 + n$; then is $x = r^z = (1 + n)^z$, and $x + \dot{x} = (1 + n)^{z + \dot{z}} = (1 + n)^z \times (1 + n)^{\dot{z}} = x \times (1 + n)^{\dot{z}}$, which by expanding $(1 + n)^{\dot{z}}$, omitting the 2d, 3d, &c powers of $\dot{z}$, and writing q for $\dfrac{n}{1 + n}$, becomes

$x + x\dot{z} \times : q + \frac{1}{2}q^2 + \frac{1}{3}q^3 + \frac{1}{4}q^4$ &c;

therefore $\dot{x} = ax\dot{z}$, putting a for the series $q + \frac{1}{2}q^2 + \frac{1}{3}q^3$ &c,

or $f\dot{x} = x\dot{z}$, putting $f = \dfrac{1}{a}$.

Now when $r = 1 + n = 10$, as in the common logarithms of Briggs's form; then $n = 9$, $q = ,9$, and the series $q + \frac{1}{2}q^2 + \frac{1}{3}q^3$ &c, gives $a = 2,302585$ &c, and therefore its reciprocal $f = ,434294$ &c. But if $a = 1 = f$, the form will be that of Napier's logarithms.

From the above form $x\dot{z} = f\dot{x}$, or $\dot{z} = \dfrac{f\dot{x}}{x}$, are then deduced many curious and general properties of logarithms, with the several series heretofore given by Gregory, Mercator, Wallis, Newton, and Halley. But of all these series, that one which our author selects for constructing the logarithms, is this, putting $N = \dfrac{r - p}{r + p}$, the logarithm of $\dfrac{r}{p}$ is $= 2f \times : N + \frac{1}{3}N^3 + \frac{1}{5}N^5 + \frac{1}{7}N^7$ &c, in the case in which $r - p$ is $= 1$, and consequently in that case $N = \dfrac{1}{2r - 1}$ or $\dfrac{1}{2p + 1}$; which series will then converge very fast.

Hence, having given any numbers, p, q, r, &c, and as many ratios a, b, c, &c, composed of them, the difference between the two terms of each ratio being 1; as also the logarithms A, B, C, &c of those ratios given: to find the logarithms P, Q, R, &c of those numbers; supposing $f = 1$. For instance, if $p = 2$, $q = 3$, $r = 5$; and $a = \dfrac{9}{8} = \dfrac{3^2}{2^3}$, $b = \dfrac{16}{15} = \dfrac{2^4}{3.5}$, $c = \dfrac{25}{24} = \dfrac{5^2}{3.2^3}$. Now the logarithms A, B, C, of these ratios a, b, c, being found by the above series, from the nature of powers we have these three equations,

$$\left.\begin{array}{l} A = 2Q - 3P \\ B = 4P - Q - R \\ C = 2R - Q - 3P \end{array}\right\} \text{which equations reduced give} \left\{\begin{array}{l} P = 3A + 4B + 2C = \text{log. of 2.} \\ Q = 5A + 6B + 3C = \text{log. of 3.} \\ R = 7A + 9B + 5C = \text{log. of 5.} \end{array}\right.$$

And hence $P + R = 10A + 13B + 7C$ is $=$ the logarithm of 2×5 or 10.

An elegant tract on logarithms, as a comment on Dr. Halley's method, was also given by Mr. Jones, in his *Synopsis Palmariorum Matheseos*, published in the year 1706. And, in the Philosophical Transactions, he communicated various improvements in goniometrical properties, and the series relating to the circle and to trigono-metry.

The memoir above described was delivered to the Royal Society by their then librarian, Mr. John Robertson, a worthy, ingenious, and industrious man; who also communicated to the Society several little tracts of his own relating to logarithmical subjects; he was also the author of an excellent Treatise on the Elements of Naviga-tion in two volumes; and he was successively mathematical master to Christ's hospital in London; to the royal naval academy at Portsmouth; and librarian, clerk, and house-keeper to the Royal Society; at whose house, in Crane-Court, Fleet-Street, he died in 1776, aged 64 years.

And among the papers of Mr. Robertson, I have, since his death, found one containing the following particulars relating to Mr. Jones, which I here insert, as I know of no other account of his life, &c, and as any true anecdotes of such extraordinary men must always be acceptable to the learned. This paper is not in Mr. Robertson's hand writing, but in a kind of running law-hand, and is signed R. M. 12 Sept. 1771.

" William Jones, Esq. F. R. S. was born at the foot of Bodavon mountain [Mynydd Bodafon], in the parish of Llansihangel tre'r Bardd, in the isle of Anglesey, North Wales, in the year 1675. His father John George * was a farmer of a good family, being descended from Hwfa ap Cynddelw, one of the fifteen tribes of North Wales. He gave his two sons the common school education of the country, reading, writing, and accounts, in English, and the Latin grammar. Harry his second son took to the farming business; but William the eldest, having an extraordinary turn for mathematical studies, determined to try his fortune abroad from a place where the same was but of little service to him; he accordingly came to Lon-don, accompanied by a young man, Rowland Williams, afterwards an eminent perfumer in Wych-Street. The report in the country is, that Mr. Jones soon got into a merchant's counting-house, and so gained the esteem of his master, that he gave him the command of a ship for a West-India voyage; and that upon his return he set up a mathematical school, and published his book of navigation †; and that upon the death of the merchant he married his widow : that Lord Macclesfield's son being his pupil, he was made secretary to the chancellor, and one of the D. tellers of exchequer—and they have a story of an Italian wedding which caused great disturbance in Lord Macclesfield's family, but compromised by Mr. Jones; which

---

* " It is the custom in several parts of Wales for the name of the father to become the sur-name of his children. John George the father was commonly called Sion Siors of Llambabo, to which parish he moved, and where his children were brought up."

† This tract on navigation, entitled, " A new Compendium of the whole Art of Practical Navigation," was published in 1702, and dedicated " to the reverend and learned Mr. John Harris, M. A. and F. R. S." the author, I apprehend, of the " Universal Dictionary of Arts and Sciences," under whose roof Mr. Jones says he composed the said treatise on Navi-gation.

R

gave rise to a saying, that Macclesfield was the making of Jones, and
Jones the making of Macclesfield."

. Mr. Jones died July 3, 1749, being vice-president of the Royal
Society : and left one daughter, and a son, born in 1748, who was the
late Sir William Jones, one of the judges in India, and highly esteemed
for his great abilities and extensive learning; and who died in India,
in the year 1794.

Euler's method given in his Introd. in Anal. Infinit. is much the
same, in manner and effect, as that of Mr. Jones, given above.

Of Mr. Andrew Reid and Others.

Andrew Reid, Esq. published in 1767 a quarto tract, under the
title of *An Essay on Logarithms*, in which he also shows the computation of logarithms from principles depending on the binomial theorem and the nature of the exponents of powers, the logarithms of
numbers being here considered as the exponents of the powers of 10.
He hence brings out the usual series for logarithms, and largely
exemplifies Dr. Halley's most simple construction.

Besides the authors whose methods have been here particularly
described, many others have treated on the subject of logarithms, and
of the sines, tangents, secants, &c; among the principal of whom
are Leibnitz, Euler, Maclaurin, Wolfius, and professor Simson in
an elegant geometrical tract on logarithms, contained in his posthumous works, elegantly printed in 4to. at Glasgow, in the year 1776,
at the expense of the very learned Earl Stanhope, and by his Lord-
ship disposed of in presents among gentlemen most eminent for mathematical learning.

Of Mr. Dodson's Anti-logarithmic Canon.

The only remaining considerable work of this kind published, that
I know of, is the Anti-logarithmic Canon of Mr. James Dodson, an
ingenious mathematician, and sometime master of the Royal Mathematical School, in Christ's Hospital, London: which work he published in folio in the year 1742 : a very great performance, containing
all logarithms under 100000, and their corresponding natural numbers
to 11 places of figures, with all their differences and the proportional
parts; the whole arranged in the order contrary to that used in the
common tables of numbers and logarithms, the exact logarithms being
here placed first, and increasing continually by 1, from 1 to 100000,
with their corresponding nearest numbers in the columns opposite to
them; and by means of the differences and proportional parts, the
logarithm to any number, or the number to any logarithm, each to
11 places of figures, is readily found. This work contains also, besides the construction of the natural numbers to the given logarithms,
" precepts and examples, showing some of the uses of logarithms,
in facilitating the most difficult operations in common arithmetic,
cases of interest, annuities, mensuration, &c; to which is prefixed
an introduction, containing a short account of logarithms, and of
the most considerable improvements made, since their invention, in the
manner of constructing them."

The manner in which these numbers were constructed, consists chiefly in imitations of some of the methods before described by Briggs, and is nothing more than generating a scale of 100000 geometrical proportionals, from 1 the least term to 10 the greatest, each continued to 11 places of figures; and the means of effecting this, are such as easily flow from the nature of a series of proportionals, and are briefly as follow. First, between 1 and 10, are interposed 9 mean proportionals; then between each of these 11 terms there are interposed 9 other means, making in all 101 terms; then between each of these a 3d set of 9 means, making in all 1001 terms; again between each of these a 4th set of 9 means, making in all 10001 terms; and lastly, between each two of these terms, a 5th set of 9 means, making in all 100001 terms, including both the 1 and the 10. The first four of these 5 sets of means, are found each by one extraction of the 10th root of the greater of the two given terms, which root is the least mean, and then multiplying it continually by itself according to the number of terms in the section or set; and the 5th or last section is made by interposing each of the 9 means by help of the method of differences before taught. Namely, putting 10 the greatest term

$= A$, $A^{\frac{1}{10}} = B$, $B^{\frac{1}{10}} = C$, $C^{\frac{1}{10}} = D$, $D^{\frac{1}{10}} = E$, and $E^{\frac{1}{10}} = F$; now extracting the 10th root of A or 10, it gives $1{,}2589254118 = B = A^{\frac{1}{10}}$ for the least of the 1st set of means; and then multiplying it continually by itself, we have B, B^2, B^3, B^4, &c, to $B^{10} = A$, for all the 10 terms: 2dly, the 10th root of $1{,}2589254118$ gives $1{,}0232929923 = C = B^{\frac{1}{10}} = A^{\frac{1}{100}}$, for the least of the 2d class of means, which being continually multiplied gives C, C^2, C^3, &c, to $C^{100} = B^{10} = A$ for all the 2d class of 100 terms: 3dly, the 10th root of $1{,}0232929923$ gives $1{,}0023052381 = D = C^{\frac{1}{10}} = B^{\frac{1}{100}} = A^{\frac{1}{1000}}$ for the least of the 3d class of means, which being continually multiplied, gives D, D^2, D^3, &c, to $D^{1000} = C^{100} = B^{10} = A$ for the 3d class of 1000 terms: 4thly, the 10th root of $1{,}0023052381$ gives $1{,}0002302850 = E = D^{\frac{1}{10}} = C^{\frac{1}{100}} = B^{\frac{1}{1000}} = A^{\frac{1}{10000}}$ for the least of the 4th class of means, which being continually multiplied, gives E, E^2, E^3, &c, to $E^{10000} = D^{1000} = C^{100} = B^{10} = A$ for the 4th class of 10000 terms. Now these 4 classes of terms, thus produced, require no less than 11110 multiplications of the least means by themselves: which however are much facilitated by making a small table of the first 10 or even 100 products of the constant multiplier, and from thence only taking out the proper lines and adding them together: and these 4 classes of numbers always prove themselves at every 10th term, which must always agree with the corresponding successive terms of the preceding class. The remaining 5th class is constructed by means of differences, being much easier than the method of continual multiplication, the 1st and 2d differences only being used, as the 3d difference is too small to enter the computation of the sets of 9 means between each two terms of the 4th class.

And the several 2d differences for each of these sets of 9 means, are found from the properties of a set of proportionals $1, r, r^2, r^3$, &c, as disposed in the 1st column of the annexed table, and their several orders of differences as in the other columns of the table; where it is evident that each column, both

Terms	1st dif.	2d dif.	3d dif.	&c
$1 \times$	$(r-1)\times$	$(r-1)^2\times$	$(r-1)^3\times$	
1	1	1	1	
r	r	r	r	&c.
r^2	r^2	r	r^2	
r^3	r^3	r,	r^3	
&c.	&c.	&c.	&c	

that of the given terms of the progression, and those of their orders of differences, forms a scale of proportionals, having the same common ratio r, and that each horizontal line, or row, forms a geometrical progression, having all the same common ratio $r-1$, which is also the 1st difference of each set of means; so $(r-1)^2$ is the 1st of the 2d differences, and which is constantly the same, as the 3d differences become too small in the required terms of our progression to be regarded, at least near the beginning of the table: hence, like as 1, $r-1$, and $(r-1)^2$ are the first term, with its 1st and 2d differences; so r^n, $r^n(r-1)$, and $r^n(r-1)^2$, are any other term with its 1st and 2d differences. And by this rule the 1st and 2d differences are to be found for every set of 9 means, viz, multiplying the 1st term of any class (which will be the several terms of the series E, E^2, E^3, &c, or every 10th term of the series F, F^2, F^3, &c), by $r-1$ or $F-1$ for the 1st difference, and this multiplied by $F-1$ again, for the true 2d difference at the beginning of that class. Thus, the 10th root of $1,0002302850$ or E gives $1,000023026116$ for F, or the 1st mean of the lowest class, therefore $F-1 = r-1 = ,000023026116$ is its 1st difference, and the square of it is $(r-1)^2 = ,0000000005302$ its 2d difference; then is $,000023026116 F^{10n}$ or $,000023026116 E^n$ the 1st difference, and $,0000000005302 F^{20n}$ or $0000000005302 E^{2n}$ is the 2d difference at the beginning of the nth class of decades. And this 2d difference is used as the constant 2d difference through all the 10 terms, except towards the end of the table, where the differences increase fast enough to require a small correction of the 2d difference, which Mr. Dodson effects by taking a mean 2d difference among all the 2d differences, in this manner; having found the series of 1st differences $(F-1)E^n$, $(F-1)E^{n+1}$, $(F-1)E^{n+2}$, &c, take the differences of these, and $\frac{1}{10}$ of them will be the mean 2d differences to be used, namely, $\frac{F-1}{10}(E^{n+1}-E)^n$, $\frac{F-1}{10}(E^{n+2}-E^{n+1})$, &c, are the mean 2d differences. And this is not only the more exact, but also the easier way. The common 2d difference, and the successive 1st differences, are then continually added, through the whole decade, to give the successive terms of the required progression.

DESCRIPTION AND USE

OF

LOGARITHMIC TABLES.

THOUGH the nature and construction of logarithms have been pretty fully treated in the preceding history of such numbers, where the more learned and curious reader will find abundant satisfaction, I shall here give a brief, easy, and familiar idea of these matters, for the practical use of young students in this subject.

The Definition and Notation of Logarithms.

Logarithms may be considered the indices or arithmetical series of numbers, adapted to the terms of a geometrical series, in such sort that 0 corresponds to 1, or is the index of it, in the geometricals.

Thus $\begin{cases} 0 & 1 & 2 & 3 & 4 & 5, \text{&c, indices or logarithms,} \\ 1 & 2 & 4 & 8 & 16 & 32, \text{&c, geometric progression.} \end{cases}$

or $\begin{cases} 0 & 1 & 2 & 3 & 4 & 5, \text{&c, indices or logarithms,} \\ 1 & 3 & 9 & 27 & 81 & 243, \text{&c, geometric series.} \end{cases}$

or $\begin{cases} 0 & 1 & 2 & 3 & 4 & 5, \text{&c, indices or logarithms,} \\ 1, & 10, & 100, & 1000, & 10000, & 100000, \text{&c, geometric series.} \end{cases}$

Where the same indices serve equally for any geometric series; and from which it is evident, that there may be an endless variety of systems of logarithms to the same common numbers, by varying the 2d term, 2, or 3, or 10, &c, of the geometric series; as this will change the original series of terms, whose indices are the integer numbers, 1, 2, 3, &c; then by interpolation the whole system of numbers may be made to enter the geometrical series, and receive their proportional logarithms, whether integers or decimals.

Or, the logarithm of any number is the index of that power of some other number, which is equal to the given number. So, if N be $= r^n$, then the logarithm of N is n, which may be either positive or negative, and r any number whatever, according to the different systems of logarithms. When N is 1, then $n=0$, whatever the value of r is; and consequently the logarithm of 1 is always 0 in every system of logarithms. When n is $= 1$, then N is $= r$: consequently r is always the number whose logarithm is 1, in every system. When r is $= 2.718281828459$ &c, the indices are the hyperbolic logarithms, such as in our 7th table: so that n is the hyperbolic logarithm of $(2.718 \text{ &c})^n$. But in the common logarithms, r

is $= 10$; so that the common logarithm of any number (10^n) is (n) the index of that power of 10 which is equal to the said number. So 1000, being the 3d power of 10, has 3 for its logarithm; and if 50 be $= 10^{1\cdot69897}$, then is $1\cdot69897$ the common logarithm of 50. And hence it follows, that this decupal series of terms

$$10^4, 10^3, 10^2, 10^1, 10^0, 10^{-1}, 10^{-2}, 10^{-3}, 10^{-4},$$

or 10000, 1000, 100, 10, 1, $\cdot1$, $\cdot01$, $\cdot001$, $\cdot0001$,

have 4, 3, 2, 1, $0, -1, -2, -3, -4$,

respectively for their logarithms.

The logarithm of a number comprehended between any two terms of the first series, is included between the two corresponding terms of the latter, and therefore that logarithm will consist of the same index (whether positive or negative) as the less of those two terms, together with a decimal fraction, which will always be positive. So the number 50, falling between 10 and 100, its logarithm will fall between 1 and 2, and is $= 1\cdot69897$, the index of the less term, together with the same decimal $\cdot 69897$ as before: also the number $\cdot05$, falling between the terms $\cdot1$ and $\cdot01$, its logarithm will fall between -1 and -2, and is indeed $= -2 + \cdot69897$, the index of the less term together with still the same decimal $\cdot69897$. The index is also called the characteristic of the logarithms, and is always an integer, either positive or negative, or else $= 0$; and it shows what place is occupied by the first significant figure of the given number, either above or below the place of units, being in the former case $+$ or positive, in the latter $-$ or negative.

When the characteristic of a logarithm is negative, the sign $-$ is commonly set over it, to distinguish it from the decimal part, which being the logarithm found in the tables, is always positive: so $-2 + \cdot69897$, or the logarithm of $\cdot05$, is written thus $\overline{2}\cdot69897$. But on some occasions it is convenient to reduce the whole expression to a negative form; which is done by making the characteristic figure less by 1, and taking the arithmetical complement of the decimal, that is, beginning at the left hand, subtract each figure from 9, except the last significant figure, which subtract from 10; so shall the remainders form the logarithm entirely negative. Thus the logarithm of $\cdot05$, which is $\overline{2}\cdot69897$, or $-2 + \cdot69897$, is also expressed by $-1\cdot30103$, which is wholly negative. It is also sometimes thought more convenient to express such logarithms wholly as positive, namely, by only joining to the tabular decimal the complement of the index to 10: in which way the above logarithm is expressed by $8\cdot69897$; which is only increasing the indices in the scale by 10. It is also convenient, in many operations with logarithms, to take their arithmetical complements, which is done, as above mentioned, by beginning at the left hand, and subtracting every figure from 9, but the last figure from 10: so the arithmetical complement

of $1\cdot69897$ $\{$and of $\overline{2}\cdot69897$ $\}$ where the index -2, being negative, is $8\cdot30103$ $\{$ it is $11\cdot30103$ $\}$ is added to 9, and makes 11.

The Properties of Logarithms.

From the definition of logarithms, either as being the indices of a series of geometricals, or as the indices of the powers of the same root, it follows, that the multiplication of the numbers will answer to the addition of their logarithms; the division of numbers, to the subtraction of their logarithms; the raising of powers, to the multiplying the logarithm of the root by the index of the power; and the extracting of roots, to the dividing the logarithm of the given number by the index of the root required to be extracted. So

1st. L. ab or $a \times b$ is $=$ L. $a +$ L. b
  L. 18 or 3×6 is $=$ L. $3 +$ L. 6
  L. $5 \times 9 \times 73$ is $=$ L. $5 +$ L. $9 +$ L. 73

2d. L. $a \div b$ is $=$ L. $a -$ L. b
  L. $18 \div 6$ is $=$ L. $18 -$ L. 6
  L. $79 \times 5 \div 9$ is $=$ L. $79 +$ L. $5 -$ L. 9
  L. $\frac{1}{2}$ or $1 \div 2$ is $=$ L. $1 -$ L. $2 = 0 -$ L. $2 = -$ L. 2

  L. $\frac{1}{n}$ or $1 \div n$ is $= -$ L. n.

3d. L. r^n is $= n$ L. r; L. $r^{\frac{1}{n}}$ or L. $\sqrt[n]{r}$ is $= \frac{1}{n}$ L. r; L. $r^{\frac{m}{n}}$ is $= \frac{m}{n}$ L. r.

  L. 2^6 is $= 6$ L. 2; L. $2^{\frac{1}{3}}$ or L. $\sqrt[3]{2}$ is $= \frac{1}{3}$ L. 2; L. $2^{\frac{2}{3}}$ is $= \frac{2}{3}$ L. 2.

So that any number and its reciprocal have the same logarithm but with contrary signs; and the sum of the logarithms of any number and its complement, is equal to 0.

To construct Logarithms.

It has been shown, in the foregoing historical part, that the logarithm of $\frac{b}{a}$ is $= \frac{2}{m} \times : \frac{x}{z} + \frac{x^3}{3z^3} + \frac{x^5}{5z^5} + \frac{x^7}{7z^7}$ &c, where z is the sum and x the difference of a and b; also $m = 2\cdot302585092994$ &c, the hyp. logarithm of 10. Therefore if a and b be any two numbers differing only by unity, so that x or $b - a$ may be $= 1$; then shall the logarithm of b be $=$ L. $a + \frac{2}{m} \times : \frac{1}{z} + \frac{1}{3z^3} + \frac{1}{5z^5}$ &c.

Which gives this rule in words at length: call z the sum of any number (whose logarithm is sought) and the number next less by unity: divide $\cdot8685889638$ &c (or $2 \div 2\cdot3025$ &c) by z, and reserve the quotient: divide the reserved quotient by the square of z, and reserve this quotient: divide this last quotient also by the square of z, and again reserve this quotient: and thus proceed continually, dividing the last quotient by the square of z, as long as division can be made. Then write these quotients orderly under one another, the first uppermost, and divide them respectively by the uneven numbers 1, 3, 5, 7, 9, 11, &c, as long as division can be made:

that is, divide the first reserved quotient by 1, the 2d by 3, the 3d by 5, the 4th by 7, &c. Add all these last quotients together, then the sum will be the logarithm of $b \div a$; and therefore to this logarithm adding also the logarithm of a the next less number, the sum will be the required logarithm of b the number proposed.

Ex. 1. *To find the Log. of 2.*

Here the next less number is 1, and $2 + 1 = 3 = z$, whose square is 9. Then

3) ·868588964 | 1)·289529654(·289529654
9)·289529654 | 3) 32169962(107233215
9) 32169962 | 5) 3574440(714888
9) 3574440 | 7) 397160(56737
9) 397160 | 9) 44129(4903
9) 44129 |11) 4903(446
9) 4903 |13) 545(42
9) 545 |15) 61(4
9) 61 | Log. ½ - ·301029995
| Add L. 1 - ·000000000
| Log. of 2 - ·301029995

Ex. 2. *To find the Log. of 3.*

Here the next less number is 2, and $2 + 3 = 5 = z$, whose square is 25, to divide by which always multiply by ·04. Then

5)·868588964 | 1)·173717793(·173717793
25)·173717793 | 3) 6948712(2316237
25) 6948712 | 5) 277948(55590
25) 277948 | 7) 11118(1588
25) 11118 | 9) 448(50
25) 445 |11) 18(2
| 18
| L. ½ - - ·176091260
| L. 2 add - ·301029995
| L. 3 - - ·477121255

Then because the sum of the logarithms of numbers gives the logarithm of their product, and the difference of the logarithms gives the logarithm of the quotient of the numbers, from the above two logarithms, and the logarithm of 10 which is 1, we may raise a great many other logarithms, thus:

Ex. 3. Because $2 \times 2 = 4$, therefore

to L. 2 - - - ·3010299954
add L. 2 - - ·3010299954
sum is L. 4 - - ·6020599914

Ex. 4. Because $2 \times 3 = 6$, therefore

to L. 2 - - - ·301029995
add L. 3 - - ·477121255
sum is L. 6 - - ·7781511250

Ex. 5. Because $2^3 = 8$, therefore

L. 2 - - - - ·3010299954
mult. by 3 - - 3
gives L. 8 - - ·903089987

Ex. 6. Because $3^2 = 9$, therefore

L. 3 - - - ·4771212547/16
mult. by 2 - 2
gives L. 9 - ·954242509

Ex. 7. Because $\frac{10}{2} = 5$, therefore

from L. 10 - 1·000000000
take L. 2 - - ·3010299954
leaves L. 5 - ·6989700044

Ex. 8. Because $12 = 3 \times 4$, therefore

to L. 3 - - - ·477121255
add L. 4 - - ·602059991
gives L. 12 - 1·079181246

And thus, computing, by the general rule, the logarithms of the other prime numbers, 7, 11, 13, 17, 19, 23, &c; and then using composition and division, we may easily find as many logarithms as we please, or may speedily examine any logarithm in the table.

THE DESCRIPTION AND USE OF THE TABLES.

THE following collection consists of various tables, in the following order, viz. 1, A large table of logarithms to 7 places of figures; 2, A table for finding logarithms and numbers to 20 places; 3, Logarithms to 20 places, with their 1st, 2d, and 3d differences; 4, Another table of logarithms to 20 places, with their 1st, 2d, and 3d differences; 5, Logarithms to 61 places; 6, Another table of logarithms to 61 places, with their 1st, 2d, 3d, and 4th differences; 7, Hyperbolic logarithms; 8, Logistic logarithms; 9, Logarithmic sines and tangents to every second of the first 2 degrees; 10, Natural and logarithmic sines, tangents, secants, and versed sines, with their differences to every minute of the quadrant. After which follow several smaller tables; as a table of the lengths of circular arcs; a traverse table, or table of difference of latitude and departure, to every degree and quarter point of the compass; a table for changing the common logarithms into hyperbolic logarithms; and a table of the names and number of degrees &c in every point of the compass; as also lists of errata in various works of this sort. Of each of which in their order.

Of the large Table of Logarithms.

The first is the large table of logarithms, to all numbers from 1 to 100000; by which may be found the logarithm to any number, and the number to any logarithm, to 7 places of figures. This table consists of two parts; the first contains, in 4 pages, the first 1000 numbers, with their corresponding logarithms in adjacent columns; the second contains all the 100000 numbers and their logarithms, with the differences and proportional parts, disposed as follows: in the 1st column of each page are the first 4 figures of the numbers, and along the top and bottom of the columns is the 5th figure, in which columns are placed all the logarithms, the first 3 figures of each logarithm being at the beginning of the lines in the first column of logarithms, signed 0 at the top and bottom, and the other 4 figures in the remaining columns. Sometimes the first three figures of the logarithms are found in the line next below the number, viz. when the fourth figures have changed from 9's to 0's, in which case, a bar is placed over the first cipher, to catch the eye, thus 0. After the 10 columns of logarithms, stands their column of differences, signed D; and lastly, after that, the column of proportional parts, signed Pro. Pts. showing what proportional part of each difference corresponds to 1, 2, 3, &c, the whole difference answering to 10; or showing the $\frac{1}{10}$, $\frac{2}{10}$, $\frac{3}{10}$, &c, of the differences.

Note, The logarithms in these columns are all supposed to be decimals, and their corresponding natural numbers may be either integers or decimals or mixt numbers; for the same figures, whatever be their denomination, have the same decimal logarithm, and these differ only in the index or characteristic, which is the integer num-

S

ber to be prefixed to the decimal part of the logarithm; and this is always the number which expresses the distance of the highest denomination, or left-hand figure, of the natural number, from the units place. So that if the natural number consist of only one place of integers, the index of its log. will be 0: if of 2, 3, 4, 5, &c, the index of its logarithm will be respectively 1, 2, 3, 4, &c, being 1 less than the number of integer places: and the same figures made negative will give the index of the logarithm of a decimal, viz. if the natural number be a decimal, and its first significant figure be in the place of primes, 2ds, 3ds, 4ths, &c, the index of its logarithm will be respectively $\overline{1}, \overline{2}, \overline{3}, \overline{4}$, &c, or the figure which expresses the distance of the first place of the natural number from the units place, but with a negative sign, as the number is below the place of units, the sign being written above the index instead of before it, as that part only of the logarithms is to be considered as negative, the decimal part of it being always affirmative. And in the arithmetical operations of addition and subtraction with logarithms, the negative indexes will have the contrary effect to that of the decimal part of the logarithm, viz. when the logarithm is to be added, the figure of the negative index must be subtracted, *et vice versa.* Hence if 4234097 be the tabular or decimal part of the logarithm belonging to the figures 2651, without any regard to their particular denominations; then according as they are varied with respect to the number of decimals, as in the 1st annexed column, the index of their logarithm, and the complete logarithm, will vary as in the 2d column here annexed. And hence, like as when the natural number is given, we find the index

Number	Logar.
2651	3·4234097
265·1	2·4234097
26·51	1·4234097
2·651	0·4234097
·2651	$\overline{1}$·4234097
·02651	$\overline{2}$·4234097
·002651	$\overline{3}$·4234097

of its logarithm by counting how far its first figure on the left hand is from the units place; so when a logarithm is given, the denominations of the figures in its natural number will be found by placing the decimal point so, that the number of integer places may be 1 more than that of the index when positive, or by setting the first significant figure in that decimal place, which is expressed by the number of the index when negative.

Of finding the Logarithm of a given Number, or the Number to a given Logarithm.

1. To find the Logarithm of a Number consisting of 3 figures.

Find the number in the column of numbers in one of the first 4 pages of the table, and immediately on the right of it is its logarithm sought. So the logarithm of 72 is 1·8573325, and the logarithm of 3·33 is 0·5224442, when the proper index is supplied.

2. *To find the Logarithm of a Number consisting of 4 Places.*

In the first column (signed N) in some one of the pages of the table after the first four, find the given number, then against it in the 2d column (signed 0) is the logarithm sought. So the logarithm of 2254 is 3·3529539, and that of 31·32 is 1··1958218.

3. *To find the Logarithm of a Number consisting of 5 Places.*

Find the first 4 figures of the given number in the first column as before, and the 5th figure at the top or bottom; then the 7 figures of the logarithm are found in two columns on the line of the first 4 figures of the given number, viz. the first 3 figures of the logarithm are the first 3 common figures of the 2d column (signed 0), and the last 4 figures are on the same line, but in the column signed with the 5th-figure of the given number. So the logarithm of 23204 is 4·3655629, and that of 746·40 is 2·8729716, and that of ·083178 is 2·9200085.

Note, When the last four figures of the logarithm begin with a cipher, or any figure less than the last four in the 2d column begins with, then the first 3 common figures are those in the next lower line: so in the last example the first 3 common figures are 920, and not 919.

4. *To find the Logarithm of a Number of 6 Places.*

Find the logarithm of the first 5 figures by the last article, and take the difference between that logarithm and the next following logarithm, or (which is the same thing) find the difference nearest opposite in the last column but one, signed D; then under that difference in the last column (of proportional parts) and against the 6th figure of the given number, is the part to be added to the logarithm before found for the first 5 figures, the sum being the logarithm sought. So to find the logarithm of 3409·26: the logarithm of 34092, the first 5 figures, being 5326525, and the common difference 127, under which and against 6 in the last column is 76, which being added to the former logarithm, and the proper index prefixed, we have 3·5326601 for the whole logarithm required.

5. *To find the Logarithm of a Number of 7 Places.*

Find the logarithm of the first 5 figures by the 3d article, and of the sixth figure by the 4th article; then for the logarithm of the 7th figure, divide its proportional part by 10, that is, set it one place farther to the right hand than the last figure of the logarithm reaches; add all the three together, and their sum will be the logarithm required.

Thus, to find the logarithm of 3·409264.

The several parts being taken out according to the rule, and placed as in the margin, the sum gives the whole logarithm sought.

Numb.	Logar.
34092 - -	5326525
6 -	76
4 -	5,1
3·409264 -	0·5326606

Note, In the same way we might take out the proportional part of an 8th figure, dividing its tabular part by 100, or setting it two places farther to the right hand than the first logarithm. Or the whole proportional part for any number of figures above five, may be found at once, by multiplying the common tabular difference of the logarithms, found as before, by all the figures after the 5th, cutting off from the product as many figures as we multiply by, and adding the rest to the logarithm of the first 5 figures before found. So in the last example above, having found the common difference 127, multiplying it by 64 the last two figures, cutting off two, add the rest to the logarithm of the first 5, as in the margin.

127
64
508
762
81,28
5326525
0·5326606

For another example, suppose we wanted the logarithm of the following 8 figures 34092648. The operation by both methods will be as below.

						127	
34092 -	-	-	-	5326525		648	
6 -	-	-	-	76		1016	
4 -	-	-	5,1		508	
8 -	-	-	1,02		762	
34092648 -	-	7·5326607		82,296	
				5326525	
				7·5326607 the same as the other.	

6. *To find the Logarithm of a Vulgar Fraction, or of a Mixt Number.*

Either reduce the vulgar fraction to a decimal, and find its logarithm as above. Or else (having reduced the mixt number to an improper fraction), subtract the logarithm of the denominator from the logarithm of the numerator, and the remainder will be the logarithm of the fraction sought.

Ex. 1. To find the log. of $\frac{3}{16}$ or 0·1875.	*Ex.* 2. To find the log. of $13\frac{3}{4}$ or $\frac{55}{4}$.
From log. of 3 - - 0.4771213	From log. of 55 - - 1·7403627
Take log. of 16 - - 1·2041200	Take log. of 4 - - 0·6020600
Rem. log. of $\frac{3}{16}$ or ·1875 1·2730013	Leaves log. of $\frac{55}{4}$ or 13·75 1·1383027

7. *To find the Natural Number answering to any given Logarithm.*

Find the first 3 figures, next after the index of the given logarithm, in the second column, signed 0, and the other 4 figures on the same line in one of the nine following columns; if the figures of the logarithm be thus found exactly, then on the same line in the first column are the first four figures of the natural number, and the 5th is at the top or bottom of that column in which the last four figures of the log. were found. So to find the number answering to the logarithm 2·5890108. In pa. 63 I find the first three figures 589, and in column 6 of the line above are found the other four ·0108 (because the first three common figures are supposed to begin at that part of the line above where they are placed): then on the same line in the column of numbers stand the first four figures 388·1, and 6 at the top of the column, making in all 388·16 for the number sought; having placed the decimal point so as to make three integers, being 1 more than 2 the index of the given logarithm.

But if the given logarithm be not found exactly in the table, subtract the next less tabular logarithm from it, and look for the remainder in the proportional parts under the difference between the two tabular logarithms next less and greater than the given logarithm, and against it, or the part next less, is a 6th figure to be annexed to the five figures before found. And if the remainder be not found exactly in the proportional parts, subtract the next less part from it, and annex a cipher to this 2d remainder, then against the nearest proportional part (either greater or less) is a 7th figure to be annexed to the six before found. And that figure will be the nearest to the truth in that place, either too much or too little.

Ex. To find the number answering to the logarithm 1·2335678. The next less tab. log. is the log. of   17122 viz.   2335545

		1st rem.	133
The difference is 254	- 5 for the part		127
and the table of pro. pts. gives		2d rem.	60
	- 2 for the part	- -	51

So that the number sought is 17·12252, making two integers for the index 1.

Or the 6th and 7th figures may be found without the table of proportional parts, by dividing the first remainder by the tabular difference, annexing one cipher to the dividend for each figure to be found. So, in the last example, the remainder 133, with two ciphers annexed, being divided by the tabular difference 254, as in the margin, the quotient gives 52 for the 6th and 7th figures, the same as before. In like manner may be found the numbers to the following logarithms.

254)133,00(52
127,0
——
600
508

Logar. 1·2345678|3·7343003|1̄·0921406|2̄·3720468|4·6123004|3·2946809
Numb. 17·16200 |5·423758 |·1236348 |·02355303|40954·39 |1970·974

OF LOGARITHMICAL ARITHMETIC.

I. *Multiplication by Logarithms.*

Add together the logarithms of all the factors; then the sum is a logarithm, the natural number corresponding to which, being found in the table, will be the product required.

Observing to add, to the sum of the affirmative indices, what is carried from the sum of the decimal parts of the logarithms.

And that the difference between the affirmative and negative indices, is to be taken for the index to the logarithm of the product.

Ex. 1. To multiply 23·14 by 5·062.	*Ex.* 2. To mul. 2·581926 by 3·457291.
23·14 its log. is 1·3643634	2·581926 its log. is 0·4119438
5·062 its log. is 0·7043221	3·457291 - - - 0·5387359
Product 117·1347 - 2·0686855	Prod. 8·92647 - - 0·9506797

Ex. 3. To mult. 3·902, and 597·16, and ·0314728 all together.	*Ex.* 4. To mult. 3·586, and 2·1046, and 0·8372, and 0·0294 all together.
3·902 its log. is 0·5912873	3·586 its log. is 0.5546103
597·16 - 2·7760907	2·1046 - - 0·3231696
·0314728 - 2̄·4979353	0·8372 1̄·9228292
Prod. 73·33533 - 1·8653133	0·0294 - - 2̄·4683473
	Prod. ·1857618 - 1̄·2689564

The 2̄ cancels the 2, and the 1 to carry from the decimals is set down.

Here the 2 to carry cancels the 2̄, and there remains the 1̄ to set down.

II. *Division by Logarithms.*

From the logarithm of the dividend, subtract the logarithm of the divisor; the remainder is a logarithm, whose corresponding number will be the quotient required.

But first observe to change the sign of the index of the logarithm of the divisor, viz. from negative to affirmative, or from affirmative to negative; then take the sum of the indices if they be of the same kind, or their difference when of different kinds, with the sign of the greater, for the index to the logarithm of the quotient.

And when 1 is borrowed in the left-hand place of the decimal part of the logarithm, add it to the index of the logarithm of the divisor when that index is affirmative, but subtract it when negative; then let the index thus found be changed, and worked with as before.

Ex. 1. To divide 24163 by 4567.

Divid. 24163 its log. 4·3831509
Divis. 4567 - - 3·6596310
Quot. 5·290782 - 0·7235199

Ex. 2. To divide 37·149 by 523·76.

Divid. 37·149 its log. 1·5699471
Divis. 523·76 - - 2·7191323
Quot. ·07092752 - 2·8508148

Ex. 3. To divide ·06314 by ·007241.

Divid. ·06314 its log. 2·8003046
Divis. ·007241 - 3̄·8597985
Quot. 8·719792 - 0·9405061

Here 1 carried from the decimals to the 3̄ makes it become 2̄, which taken from the other 2̄, leaves 0 remaining.

Ex. 4. To divide ·7438 by 12·9476.

Divid. ·7438 its log. 1̄·8714562
Divis. 12·9476 - - 1·1121893
Quot. ·05744694 - 2̄·7592669

Here the 1 taken from the 1̄ makes it become 2̄ to set down.

III. *The Rule of Three, or Proportion.*

Add the logarithms of the 2d and 3d terms together, and from their sum subtract the logarithm of the 1st, by the foregoing rules; the remainder will be the logarithm of the 4th term required.

Or in any compound proportion whatever, add together the logarithms of all the terms that are to be multiplied, and from that sum take the sum of the others; the remainder will be the logarithm of the term sought.

But instead of subtracting any logarithm, we may add its complement, and the result will be the same. By the complement is meant the logarithm of the reciprocal of the given number, or the remainder by taking the given logarithm from 0 or from 10, changing the radix from 0 to 10; the easiest method of doing which, is to begin at the left-hand, and subtract each figure from 9, except the last significant figure on the right-hand, which must be subtracted from 10. But when the index is negative, add it to 9, and subtract the rest as before. And for every complement that is added, subtract 10 from the last sum of the indices.

Ex. 1. To find a 4th proportional to 72·34, and 2·519, and 357·4862.

As 72·34 - comp. log. 8·1406215
To 2·519 - - - - 0·4012282
So 357·4862 - - - 2·5532592
To 12·44827 - - - 1·0951089

Ex. 2. To find a 3d proportional to 12·796 and 3·24718.

As 12·796 - comp. log. 8·8929258
To 3·24718 - - - - 0·5115064
So 3·24718 - - - - 0·5115064
To ·8240216 - - - 1̄·9159386

Ex. 3. To find a number in proportion to ·379145 as ·85132 is to ·0649.

As ·0649 - comp. log. 11·1877553
To ·85132 - - - - 1̄·9300928
So ·379145 - - - 1̄·5788054
To 4·973401 - - - 0·6966535

Ex. 4. If the interest of 100*l.* for a year or 365 days be 4·5*l.* what will be the interest of 279·25*l.* for 274 days?

As {100}{365} comp. log. {8·0000000}{7·4377071}
To {279·25 - - - 2·4459932}{274 - - - 2·4377506}
So 4·5 - - - - 0·6532125
To 9·433296 - - - 0·9746634

IV. *Involution, or Raising of Powers.*

Multiply the logarithm of the number given by the proposed index of the power, and the product will be the logarithm of the power sought.

Note, In multiplying a logarithm with a negative index by any affirmative number, the product will be negative.—But what is to be carried from the decimal part of the logarithm will be affirmative.—Therefore the difference will be the index of the product; and it is to be accounted of the same kind with the greater.

Ex. 1. To find the 2d power of 2·5791.

Root 2·5791 its log. 0·4114682
index - - 2
Power 6·651756 - 0·8229364

Ex. 3. To find the 4th power of ·09163.

Root ·09163 its log. $\overline{2}$·9620377
index - - - 4
Power ·0000704938 - $\overline{5}$·8481508

Here 4 times the negative index being $\overline{8}$, and 3 to carry, the difference $\overline{5}$ is the index of the product.

Ex. 2. To find the cube of 3·07146.

Root 3·07146 its log. 0·4873449
index - - - 3
Power 28·97575 - 1·4620347

Ex. 4. To find the 365th power of 1.0045.

Root 1·0045 its log. 0·0019499
index - - 365
97495
116994
58497
Power 5·148888 - 0·7117135

V. *Evolution, or Extraction of Roots.*

Divide the logarithm of the power, or given number, by its index, and the quotient will be the logarithm of the root required.

Note, When the index of the logarithm is negative, and the divisor is not exactly contained in it without a remainder, increase it by such a number as will make it exactly divisible; and carry the units borrowed, as so many tens, to the left-hand place of the decimal part of the logarithm; then divide the results by the index of the root.

Er. 1. To find the square root of
365.

Power 365 - 2) 2·5622929
Root 19·10498 - 1·2811465

Er. 2. To find the cube root of
12345.

Power 12345 - 3) 4·0914911
Root 23·11162 - 1·3638304

Er. 3. To find the 10th root of 2.

Power 2 - - 10) 0·3010300
Root 1·071773 - 0·0301030

Er. 4. To find the 365th root of
1·045.

Power 1·045   365) 0.0191163
Root 1·000121 - 0·0000524

Er. 5. To find the square root of
·093.

Power ·093 - 2) $\bar{2}$·9684829
Root ·304959 - $\bar{1}$·4842415

Here the divisor 2 is contained exactly once in $\bar{2}$ the negative index, therefore the index of the quotient is $\bar{1}$.

Er. 6. To find the cube root of
·00048.

Power ·00048 3) $\bar{4}$·6812412
Root ·07829735 - $\bar{2}$·8937471

Here the divisor 3 not being exactly contained in $\bar{4}$, augment it by 2, to make it become $\bar{6}$, in which the divisor is contained just $\bar{2}$ times; and the 2 borrowed being carried to the other figures 6 &c, makes 2·6812412, which divided by 3 gives ·8937471.

OF THE TABLES FOR LOGARITHMS TO TWENTY PLACES.

THESE are tables 2d, 3d, and 4th, beginning at page 187. Of these, table 2 contains all numbers from 1 to 1000, and all uneven numbers from 1000 to 1161; with their logarithms to twenty places: table 3 contains all numbers from 101000 to 101139, with their logarithms to twenty places, and the 1st, 2d, and 3d differences of those logarithms: and table 4 contains all logarithms regularly from 00001 to 00139, with their corresponding natural numbers to twenty places, as also the 1st, 2d, and 3d differences of those numbers. And by means of them may be found the logarithm to any other number, and the number to any other logarithm, to twenty places of figures.

(1.) *To find the Logarithms to given Numbers.*

CASE 1. If the given number *b* be found in any of these three tables; then its logarithm B is in the line even with it.

CASE 2. If *b* is known to be the product or quotient of numbers found in these tables; then B is the sum or difference of the logarithms of those numbers.

T

CASE 3. If a', the first six significant figures of a given number b', be found in table 3; let a' be an integer, A' its logarithm; δ the remaining figures of b'; x the complement of δ to d' or 1; D', D'', D''', the 1st, 2d, 3d differences of the logarithms in the same line with A'; $f = \frac{1}{3} D''' \times \overline{x+1} + D''$: Then B' the logarithm of the number b' will be

$$\left. \begin{array}{l} D' \times \delta + A' \quad - \;-\; \text{to 12} \\ \overline{\tfrac{1}{2} x D'' + D'} \times \delta + A' \;-\quad \text{to 17} \\ \overline{\tfrac{1}{2} x f \;+ D'} \times \delta + A' \;-\;-\; \text{to 20} \end{array} \right\} \text{places of figures nearly.}$$

Ex. 1. Given the number $b' = 0\cdot01010,26227,6351$, to find B' its logarithm nearly to twelve places.

Here $a' = 101026$ $A' = \quad 00443,31579,747$

$\delta = 0\cdot2276351$ $\delta\, D' \; \ldots\ldots \quad + \;\; 9785,618-$

$D' = 429881746$ $B' = \overline{2\cdot00443,41365,365-}$

Ex. 2. Given $b' = 0\cdot01010,26227,63509,626$, to find B' its log. nearly to 17 places.   Here $a' = 101026$.

$\delta = 0\cdot22763,509626$; $x = 0\cdot772365$; $D' = 42988,174579$; $D'' = 425510$.

Now $\frac{1}{2} x\, D''$ .... $16432,45$

D' .... $42988,17457,86$

$\overline{\tfrac{1}{2} x\, D'' + D'}$ .... $42988,33890,31$

$\overline{\tfrac{1}{2} x\, D'' + D'} \times \delta$ .... $9785,65466,42$

A' .... $0\cdot0443,31579,74695,33$

And $\frac{1}{2} x\, D'' + D' \times \delta + A'$, or B' .... $\overline{2\cdot00443,41365,40161,75}$

Ex. 3. Given $b' = 0\cdot01010,26227,63509,62573,17345$, to find B' its log. nearly to 20 places. $a' = 101026$.

$\delta = 0\cdot22763,50962,573173$; $x = 0\cdot77236,490374$; $x + 1 = 1\cdot772365$; $D' = 42988,17457,86301$; $D'' = 42550,96343$; $D''' = 84236$.

Now $\frac{1}{3} D''' \times \overline{x+1}$ 49766

D'' .... $42550,96343$

f .... $42551,46109$

$\frac{1}{2} x f$ .... $16432,62757$

D' .... $42988,17457,86301$

$\overline{\tfrac{1}{2} x f + D'}$ .... $42988,33890,49058$

$\overline{\tfrac{1}{2} x f + D'} \times \delta$ .... $9785,65466,45604$

A' .... $00443,31579,74695,32791$

And B' .... $\overline{2,00443,41365,40161,78395}$

CASE 4. If the number b do not come under one of the preceding cases: put a for the first five figures of b; n for 101, the least, or some one, of the numbers in table 3; then $\frac{a}{n}$ or $\frac{n}{a} = a$ is to be had in table 2, with A its logarithm; let $b' = \frac{b}{a}$ or ba, and a' the first six significant figures of b' (found in table 3) be an integer, and A' its logarithm; put δ for the remaining figures of b'; x the complement of δ to d'; D', D'', D''', the 1st, 2d, 3d, differences of the logarithms in the same line with A'; $f = \frac{1}{2} D''' \times \overline{x + 1} + D''$. Then B the logarithm of the number b will be

$$D' \times \delta + A' \pm A = B' \pm A \text{ to } 12$$
$$\overline{\tfrac{1}{2} x D'' + D'} \times \delta + A' \pm A = B' \pm A \text{ to } 17 \left.\right\} \begin{array}{l} \text{places of} \\ \text{figures nearly.} \end{array}$$
$$\overline{\tfrac{1}{2} x f + D'} \times \delta + A' \pm A = B' \pm A \text{ to } 20$$

Ex. Given $b = 3\cdot14159{,}26535{,}89793{,}23846{,}26434$, to find B to twenty places.

Here $\alpha = 31415$ Let $a = \dfrac{\alpha}{n} = 311$.

Then $b' = \dfrac{b}{a} = 0\cdot01010{,}15840{,}95144{,}02970{,}57$; $a' = 101015$.

$\delta = 0\cdot84095{,}14402{,}97057$; $x = 0\cdot15904{,}85597$; $x + 1 = 1\cdot15905$; $D' = 42992{,}85574{,}06337$; $D'' = 42560{,}23099$; $D''' = 84263$.

Now $\frac{1}{2} D''' \times \overline{x + 1}$	32555
D''	42560,23099
f	42560,55654
$\frac{1}{2} x f$	3384,59761
D'	42992,85574,06337
$\frac{1}{2} x f + D'$	42992,88958,66098
$\frac{1}{2} x f + D' \times \delta$	36154,93242,03919
A'	00438,58681,74054,30961
A	49276,03890,26837,50555
And B	0·49714,98726,94133,85435

Or let $a = \dfrac{n}{\alpha} = 3\cdot216 = 0\cdot536 \times 6$.

Then $b' = ba = 10\cdot10336{,}19739{,}44775{,}0549$; $a' = 101033$.
$\delta = 0\cdot61973{,}94477{,}50549$; $x = 0\cdot38026{,}055225$; $x + 1 = 1\cdot38026$; $B' = 42985{,}19618{,}80760$; $D'' = 42545{,}06747$; $D''' = 84219$.

Now $\frac{1}{2} D''' \times \overline{x + 1}$	38748
D''	42545,06747
f	42545,45495
$\frac{1}{2} x f$	8089,17910
D'	42985,19618,80760
$\frac{1}{2} x f + D'$	42985,27707,98670
$\frac{1}{2} x f + D' \times \delta$	26639,67187,88811
A'	00446,32488,03359,61854
B'	1·00446,59127,70547,50665
A	0·50731,60400,76413,65230
$B = B' - A$	0·49714,98726,94133,85435

(II.) *To find the Numbers to given Logarithms.*

CASE 1. When the logarithm ʙ˙ is found in any of these three tables; then its number b is in the line even with it.

CASE 2. If the first five figures (omitting the index) of a given logarithm ʙ′, be between 00432 and 00492: take them as an integer, and put ᴀ′ and c′ for the logarithms, in table 3, next less and greater than ʙ′, a' and c' their numbers; let ᴅ′ ($= c' - $ ᴀ′) and ᴅ″ be the 1st and 2d differences in the line with ᴀ′; $\Delta = $ ʙ′ $-$ ᴀ′; $d' = (c' - a' =)$ 1; $x = \dfrac{\text{D}' - \Delta}{\text{D}'}$; $\delta = \dfrac{\Delta}{\text{D}' + \frac{1}{2} \text{x} \text{D}''}$: then $b' = a' + \delta$, nearly true to 17 places of figures.

Ex. Given the logarithm ʙ′ .... $= 5{,}00446{,}59127{,}70547{,}507$
to find b' its number.

$$\text{A}' = 5{,}00446{,}32488{,}03359{,}619$$

$a' = 101033$	$\Delta = 0\text{·}26639{,}67187{,}888$
δ .... $0\text{·}61973{,}944776$	$\text{D}' = 0\text{·}42985{,}19618{,}808$
$b' = \overline{101033\text{·}61973{,}944776}$	$\text{D}' - \Delta = 0\text{·}16345{,}52430{,}920$

$$x = 0\text{·}38026$$
$$\text{D}'' = 0\text{·}00000{,}42545$$
$$\tfrac{1}{2}\,x\,\text{D}'' = 0\text{·}00000{,}08089{,}1$$
$$\text{D}' + \tfrac{1}{2}\,x\,\text{D}'' = 0\text{·}42985{,}27707{,}9$$

But when any other logarithm ʙ is given, subduct ·004321 from the first six figures of ʙ: call the remainder ʀ, and let ᴀ be the logarithm in table 2, next less than ʀ, or next greater than the complement of ʀ, and a its number: then ʙ′ $=$ ʙ $-$ ᴀ, or ʙ′ $=$ ʙ $+$ ᴀ, will be within the limits of table 3, and b' will be found as in the preceding example; and if ʙ′ $=$ ʙ $-$ ᴀ, then $b = ab'$; or if ʙ′ $=$ ʙ $+$ ᴀ, then $b = \dfrac{b'}{a}$.

CASE 3. If ᴀ′, the first five figures (omitting the index) of a given logarithm ʙ′, be found in table 4: let a' be its number; and put ᴀ′ as an integer, and Δ the remaining figures of ʙ′, and x the complement of Δ to ᴅ′; d', d'', d''', the 1st, 2d, 3d differences of the numbers in the same line with a'; $f = d'' - \frac{1}{3} d''' \times \overline{x + 1}$: then the number b', whose logarithm is ʙ′, will be

$$\overline{d' \times \Delta + a'} \quad - - \quad \text{to } 12$$
$$\overline{d' - \tfrac{1}{2} \times d'' \times \Delta + a'} \quad - - \quad \text{to } 17$$
$$\overline{d' - \tfrac{1}{6} \times f \times \Delta + a'} \quad - \quad \text{to } 20$$

places of figures nearly.

Ex. Given the logarithm ʙ′ $= 0\text{·}00006{,}93311{,}37711{,}69929$, to find b' its number to 20 places. Here ᴀ′ $= 00006$.
$\Delta = 0\text{·}93311{,}37711{,}69929$; x $= 0\text{·}06688{,}622883$; x $+ 1 = 1\text{·}066886$;
$d' = 23029{,}29742{,}21293$; $d'' = 53027{,}52746$; $d''' = 1\text{·}22100.$

Now $\frac{1}{3} d''' \times \overline{x+1}$ 43422

d'' 53027,52746

f 53027,09324

$\frac{1}{2} x f$ 1773,39115

d' 23029,29742,21293

$d' - \frac{1}{2} x f$ 23029,27968,82178

$d' - \frac{1}{2} x f \times \Delta$ 21488,93801,72000

a' 10001,38164,64943,57474

And b' .... $1\cdot00015,96535,87452,9474$

CASE 4. If the logarithm B do not come under one of the preceding cases. Put A for the logarithm in table 2, next less than B, or next greater than the complement of B, and a its number; let $B' = B - A$, or $B' = B + A$; and A', the first five figures of B', may be had in table 4, with d' its number; put A' as an integer, and let Δ be the remaining figures of B'; x the complement of Δ to D'; d', d'', d''', the 1st, 2d, 3d differences of the numbers in the same line with a'; $f = d'' - \frac{1}{3} d''' \times \overline{x+1}$: then the number b', whose logarithm is B', will be

$$\overline{d' \times \Delta + a'} \times a = ab' \text{ to } 11$$
$$\overline{d' - \frac{1}{3} \times d'' \times \Delta + a'} \times a = ab' \text{ to } 16 \left. \right\} \text{ places of figures nearly.}$$
$$\overline{d' - \frac{1}{2} \times f \times \Delta + a'} \times a = ab' \text{ to } 19$$

Ex. Given $B = 4\cdot46372,61172,07184,15204$, to find b its number.
Let $A = 1\cdot46239,79978,98956,08733.$ $a = 29.$

$B' = B - A = 5\cdot00132,81193,08228,06471.$ $A' = 00132$
$\Delta = 0\cdot81193,08228,06471$; $x = 0\cdot18806,91772$; $x+1 = 1\cdot18807$;
$d' = 23096,20835,34589$; $d'' = 53181,59733$; $d''' = 1\cdot22457.$

Now $\frac{1}{3} d''' \times \overline{x+1}$ 48496

d'' 53181,59733

f 53181,11237

$\frac{1}{2} x f$ 5000,86402

d' 23096,20835,34589

$d' - \frac{1}{2} x f$ 23096,15834,48187

$d' - \frac{1}{2} x f \times \Delta$ 18752,48284,85771

a' 10030,44036,01963,96855

b' 10030,62788,50248,82626

$b = ab'$ .... $0\cdot00029,08882,08665,72159,6154$

Or, given B $= \overline{4}$·46372,61172,07184,15204, to find b.
Let A $=$ 2·53655,84425,71530,11205. $a = 344$.

$B' = B + A = \overline{1}$·00028,45597,78714,26409. $A' =$ 00028.

$\Delta =$ 0·45597,78714,26409; x $=$ 0·54402,21286; $\overline{x + 1} =$ 1·54402;
$d' =$ 23040,96629,91521; $d'' =$ 53054,39634; $d''' =$ 1·22163.

Now $\frac{1}{3} d''' \times \overline{x + 1}$	....	62874
d''	....	53054,39634
f	....	53053,76760
$\frac{1}{4} x f$	....	14431,21179
d'	....	23040,96629,91521
$d' - \frac{1}{4} x f$	....	23040,82198,70342
$\overline{d' - \frac{1}{4} x f} \times \Delta$	....	10506,10496,55627
a'	....	10006,44931,70511,67281
b'	....	10006,55437,81008,22908
$b = \dfrac{b'}{a}$	....	0·00029,08882,08665,72159,616

OF THE TABLES FOR LOGARITHMS TO SIXTY-ONE PLACES.

THESE are tables 5 and 6, from page 203 to page 207 ; the former containing the natural numbers in regular order from 1 to 100, and after that all the primes up to 1100, with their corresponding logarithms, to sixty-one places of figures; and the latter in page 207 contains all numbers in order from 999980 to 1000020, with their logarithms, to sixty-one places, as also the 1st, 2d, 3d, and 4th differences of these logarithms.   And the use of these tables, in finding the logarithm to any number, or the number to any logarithm, each to sixty-one places of figures, will be as follows.

1. *Any Number being given, to find its Logarithm to 61 Places of Figures.*

IF the given number be in either of the tables, its logarithm is found in the line even with it.

When the given number is the product or quotient of any two or more numbers found in the tables, the sum or difference of their logarithms is the logarithm of the given number.

When the given number is not in either table, or is not the product or quotient of any there, then divide 99999800000000 by the first six figures of the given number; the quotient, if composed by the multiplication, or division, or both, of any numbers in table 5, or the nearest number to the quotient so composed, will for the most part be a factor for multiplying the given number, to make the first six or seven figures of the product, with the residue as a decimal, near one of the numbers in table 6, whose logarithm is there given; and the logarithm of the fraction made by the product and that number (found by the series in page 109) added, if the product be the greater, or subtracted, if the less, will give the logarithm of the product; then subtracting the logarithm of the factor, the remainder is the logarithm of the given number; but if no such product can be had, then seek for some product composed of numbers in the tables, as shall have the first six, seven, or more figures thereof the same as those of the given number, or of some product of it made by one or more of the said numbers, by which its logarithm will be found as before.

Let the logarithm of (II), 3·14159,26535,89793,23846,26433,83279,50288,41971,69399,37510,58209,74944,59230 (the circumference of a circle whose diameter is 1, or the measure of the arc of 180 deg. when the radius is 1) be sought, and thereby the logarithm of (M) the measure of the arc of 1 minute.

99999800000000 divided by 314159 quotes 318310 nearly, which (being composed of 229 × 1390) is a fit multiplier for the number 3·14159 &c, whose product 1000000·35756,41670,85735,04401,53316,98363,06680,09915,15089,93387,45346, 13&c suits very well, being nearest 1000000 in table 6. But if no such product could have been found, or that it is known, the product of some others (as 313 × 271 divided by 27) will suit nearer, and shorten the operation: instead of the multiplier 318310, take 27, then the product is 84·82300, 16460,24417,43849,13713,48546,57787,33235,73783,12785,71663,23503,9921 = *b*, and the first five figures 84·823 (3·13 × 27·1) = *a*.

$$\text{Let } \frac{b-a}{b+a} = \frac{x}{z} = \cdots$$

0·00000,16460,24417,43849,13713,48546,57787,33235,73783,12785,71663,23504	= A.
169·64600,16460,24417,43849,13713,48546,57787,33235,73783,12785,71663,23504	

A .... 0·00000,00097,08006,09180,37507,16877,07959,99442,15465,88288,82125,59471,23822

⅓A³ 3,04978,24842,80129,87165,70018,85854,85088,40896

⅕A⁵ 17245,67496,58350,23735,18262

⅟₇A⁷ 1160,94659

Natural logarithm of $\dfrac{b}{a}$ ....0·00000,00097,08006,09180,37510,21855,32802,79572,10877,25804,26330,70055,86039

This multiplied by 0·86858,89638&c gives Briggs's logarithm of $\dfrac{b}{a}$.

Briggs's logarithm of $\dfrac{b}{a}$ .... 0·00000,00084,32266,95190,70452,98319,82138,06447,98123,25534,00216,080009

Log. of 3·13 .... 0·49554,43375,46448,48480,81265,04861,24315,15792,98693,98571,52993,196813

Log. of 27·1 .... 1·43296,92008,74405,72952,11801,94875,18026,90280,28099,73147,47106,059083

Sum = log. of b .... 1·92851,36368,53121,16625,63519,98056,24480,12520,64916,05253,00406,236505

Log. of 27 subtract .... 1·43136,37641,58987,31188,50837,09765,34592,76005,86592,57208,75944,805969

Log. of (II) 3·14159&c .... 0·49714,98726,94133,85435,12682,88290,89387,36516,78324,38044,24461,340536

Log. of 10800 (=log. of 180+log. of 60) subtract 4·03342,37554,86049,70231,25614,99214,33108,11367,66355,49630,46771,104518

Log. of (M) 0·00029,08882&c .... 6·46372,61172,07184,15203,87067,89076,56689,25149,11968,88413,77690,236018

Note, The index of this last logarithm being − 4, its complement (6) is set down, that it may be like those of the log. sines, tangents, &c.

2. *Any Logarithm being given, to find its corresponding Number to 61 Places of Figures.*

If the given logarithm be in either of the tables, its number is found in the same line prefixed.

If the given logarithm be not in the tables, then find the first seven or eight figures of the number by any other table of logarithms; and if six or all of them be the component of numbers in these tables, it will suit very well; but if not, the nearest number thereto, either greater or less, composed of these numbers, will do; for the logarithm of such component is had in these tables; then the number answering to the difference of the two logarithms (found by Dr. Halley's rule in page 110, for finding the number from the log. given) multiplied by that component, gives the number sought.

Let the example be to find the number represented by $\overline{1\cdot06}^{\overset{x}{783}}$, or the amount of one pound for one day, at the rate of 6*l.* *per cent.* *per ann.* compound interest.

The log. of 1·06 (= log. of 0·53 + log. of 2)... 0·02530,58652,64770,24084,67311,86351,74961,94636,92282,75704,63219,045305

$\frac{x}{783}$ of log. of 1·06 = L .... 0·00006,93311,37711,69928,09910,44346,16917,70396,26554,19933,43734,846699

To which the nearest number of six figures (found in the first or general table) answering, though greater, composed of numbers in table 5, is 1·00016 (=7·6 × 0·47 × 0·28) = *b.*

Log. of *b* (=log. of 7·6+log.of 0·47 +log. of 0·28)=0·00006,94815,58728,03751,77247,12696,73825,86672,64357,99684,49976,894931

From which subtract L .... 0·00006,93311,37711,69928,99910,44346,16917,70396,26554,19933,43734,846699

There will remain *l* .... 0·00000,01504,21016,33822,77336,68350,56908,16276,37803,79751,06242,048232

This multiplied by $m = 2·30258$ &c, produces $ml = 0·00000,03463$&c $= \text{A}.$

A	0·00000,03463,57189,89341,69713,22305,54835,82225,32861,41751,01028,013306
A²	119,96330,29908,64503,38236,86101,03636,37764,19566,537177
A³	4,15501,52514,24837,28993,16427,39396,16938,866927
A⁴	14391,19406,44779,60302,49067,81615,535389
A⁵	498,44935,35383,40809,76217,006709
A⁶	17,26415,17393,73003,838899
A⁷	5979 5,63082,412052
A⁸	2071,064666

$1 + \frac{1}{2} A^2$ .... 1·00000,00000,00059,98165,14954,32251,69118,43050,51818,18882,09783,268588

$\frac{1}{24} A^4$ 599,63308,60199,15012,60377,82567,313975

$\frac{1}{720} A^6$ 2397,79885,27184,727554

$\frac{1}{40320} A^8$ 51366

Sum of the affirmative parts .... 1·00000,00000,00059,98165,14954,32851,32427,03249,69228,59145,19535,361483

A .... 0·00000,03463,57189,89341,69713,22305,54835,82225,32861,41751,01028,013306

$\frac{1}{6} A^3$ 69250,25419,04139,54832,19404,56566,02823,144488

$\frac{1}{120} A^5$ 4,15374,46128,19506,74801,808389

$\frac{1}{5040} A^7$ 11,86421,246511

Sum of the negative parts .... 0·00000,03463,57189,89342,38963,47724,58979,52431,98394,17835,65074,212694

Result of the series .... 0·99999,96535,42870,08822,75990,85126,73447,50817,70834,41309,54461,148789 .

Which multiplied by 1·00016 gives (1·06$^{\frac{1}{365}}$) 1·00015,96535,87452,94744,17155,00980,35475,25977,83917,74660,15413,862573

¶ If it be required to find the number represented by 1·05$^{\frac{1}{365}}$, or the amount of one pound for one day at the rate of 5l. per cent. per ann. compound interest.

The log. of 1·05 (= log. of 0·21 + log. of 5) = 0·02118,92990,69938 &c, and $\frac{1}{365}$ thereof is 0·00005,80528,74164 &c, = L, to which the nearest number of eight figures answering, but less, composed of numbers in table 5, is 1·0001334(= 1·51 × 0·83 × 0·42 × 1·9) = a; this will converge swifter than the preceding. Such expedients may be found for most numbers that can be proposed.

Note, Of any number produced between the numbers in table 6, the logarithm may be most easily had to 30 places, by the several differences annexed.

OF THE TABLE OF HYPERBOLIC LOGARITHMS.

This is table 7, in pages 208 - - - 211, which contain the series of numbers 1·01, 1·02, 1·03, &c, to 10·00, with their hyperbolic logarithms to seven places of figures. They are so called because they square the asymptotic spaces of the right-angled hyperbola ; and they are very useful in finding fluents, and the sums of infinite series. The table, as well as the following rules, were first given at the end of Simpson's fluxions, but they were rendered much more correct in the French edition of Gardiner's tables, printed at Avignon in 1770, being very incorrect in the last figure in Simpson's book. But both those books are very erroneous in the example for finding logarithms by the table.

1. *When the given Number is between 1 and 10.*

From the given number subtract the next less tabular number, divide the remainder by the said tabular number increased by half the remainder; add the quotient to the logarithm of the said tabular number, and the sum will be the logarithm of the number proposed.

Ex. To find the hyperbolic logarithm of 3·45678. Here the next less number is 3·45, and its logarithm 1·2383742, the remainder or dividend ·00678, its half 339, which joined to

3·45339) ·00678 (·0019633
                1·2383742
           log. 1·2403375

the tabular number 3·45, gives the divisor; the quotient ·0019633 added to the tabular logarithm 1·2383742, gives 1·2403375 the required logarithm of 3·45678.

2. *When the given Number exceeds 10.*

Find the logarithm of the number as above, supposing all the figures after the first to be decimals, then to that logarithm add 2·3025851, or 4·6051702, or 6·9077553, &c, according as the given number contains 2, or 3, or 4, &c, places of integers. That is, add 2·302585092994 multiplied by the index of the power of 10, by which the given number was divided to bring it to one integer, or within the limits of the table.

Ex. To find the hyperbolic logarithm of 345·678. This number divided by 100 or 10^2, to bring it within the limits of the table, or removing the decimal point two places, gives 3·45678, the logarithm of which as above found is 1·2403375, to which adding 4·6051702

1·2403375
4·6051702
5·8455077

the hyperbolic logarithm of 100, the sum is 5·8455077 the hyperbolic logarithm required of 345·678.

Note, The hyperbolic logarithm of any number may be also found from Briggs's logarithms, viz. multiplying Briggs's logarithm of the same number by the hyperbolic logarithm of 10, viz.

Multiplying by - - - - 2·30258,50929,94045,68401,79914,
Or dividing by its reciprocal   ·43429,44819,03251,82765,11289.

OF THE LOGISTIC LOGARITHMS.

These are in table 8, pages 212 - - - 216, which contain the logistic logarithm of every second as far as the first 80′ or 4800″.

The logistic logarithm of any number of seconds is the difference between the logarithm of 3600″ and the logarithm of that number of seconds.

The chief use of the table of logistic logarithms, is for the ready computing a proportional part in minutes and seconds, when two terms of the proportion are minutes and seconds, hours and minutes, or other numbers.

When two terms of the proportion are common numbers, their common logarithms may be used instead of their logistic logarithms, putting the logarithm where its complement should be, and the contrary.

1. *To find the Logistic Logarithm of any Number of Minutes and Seconds, within the Limits of the Table.*

At the top of the table find the minutes, and in the same column, even with the seconds on the left-hand side, is the logistic logarithm.

Note, When hours are made any terms of the proportion, they are to be taken as if they were minutes, and the minutes of an hour as if they were seconds.

2. *To find the Logistic Logarithm of any Number not exceeding 4800.*

In the 2d row, next the top of the table, find the number next less than that given; then in the same column, even with the difference on the left-hand side, is found the logistic logarithm.

When two given terms of the proportion are common numbers, one or both greater than 4800, take their halves, thirds, &c, instead of them. But when only one of the given terms is a common number, and that greater than 4800, take its half, third, &c, and multiply the 4th term by 2, 3, &c.

The logistic logarithms in this table are all affirmative, as well above as below 60′; but the index of those above 60′ is − 1; below 60′ down to 6′, the index is 0; and below 6′, the indices (being either 1, 2, or 3) are expressed in the table.

U 2

EXAMPLES.

As 60′	- - lo. log.	As 60′	- - lo. log.	As 60′	- - lo. log.
To 46′ 12″	- 0·1135	To 78′ 27″	- 1·8836	To 1531	- 0·3713
So 8 7	- 0·8688	So 13 53	- 0·6357	So 40′ 12″	- 0·1135
To 6 15	- 0·9823	To 18 9	- 0·5193	To 1179	- 0·4848

As 46′ 12″	co. 1·8865	As 78′ 27″	co. 0·1164	As 40′ 12″	co. 1·8865
To 60 0	- 0·0000	To 60 0	- 0·0000	To 1179	- 0·4848
So 6 15	- 0·9823	So 18 9	- 0·5193	So 60′ 0″	- 0·0000
To 8 7	- 0·8688	To 13 53	- 0·6357	To 1531	- 0·3713

As 60′	- co. 0·0000	As 24ʰ	co. 1·6021	As 24ʰ	co. 1·6021
To 4721	- 1·8823	To 46′ 11″	- 0·1137	To 76′ 34″	- 1·8941
So 37′ 28″	- 0·2045	So 8ʰ 7′	- 0·8688	So 13ʰ 53′	- 0·6357
To 2948	- 0·0868	To 15′ 37″	- 0.5846	To 44′ 17″	- 0·1319

As 4721	- co. 0·1177	As 46′ 11″	co. 1·8863	As 76′ 34″	co. 0·1059
To 60′ 0″	- 0·0000	To 24ʰ	- 0·3979	To 24ʰ	- 0·3979
So 2948	- 0·0868	So 15′ 37″	- 0·5846	So 44′ 17″	- 0·1319
To 37′ 28″	- 0·2045	To 8ʰ 7′	- 0·8688	To 13ʰ 53′	- 0·6357

The logistic logarithms may conveniently be used in trigonometrical operations, when two of the terms are small arcs, with the logarithmic sines or tangents of other arcs; observing, that instead of the logarithmic sine or tangent, to take the complement of their logistic logarithm; and the contrary.

But this may be as readily and more naturally done by the logarithmic sines and tangents themselves of such small arcs, as taken from the next following table of sines and tangents for every second of the first 2° or 120′,

OF THE LOGARITHMIC SINES AND TANGENTS TO EVERY SECOND.

Table 9, pages 218 - - - 247, contains the log. sines and tangents for every single second of the first 2 degrees of the quadrant; the sines being placed on the left-hand pages, and the tangents on the right. The degrees and minutes are placed at the top of the columns, and the seconds on the left-hand side, of each page, the logarithmic sine or tangent being found in the common angle of meeting. So of 1° 52′ 54″ the log. sine is 8·5163420, and the log. tangent 8·5165762.

The same numbers are also the cosines and cotangents of the last 2 degrees of the quadrant, those degrees with their minutes being placed at the bottom of the columns, and their seconds ascending on the right-hand side of the pages. So the cosine of 88° 7' 6'' is 8·5163420, and its contangent 8·5165762.

When it is required to find the sine or tangent &c to 3ds &c, or any other fractional part of a second, subtract the tabular sine or tangent of the complete seconds from the next to it in the table, and take the like proportional part of the difference; which part added to, or taken from, the said tabular sine or tangent, according as it is increasing or decreasing, will give the sine or tangent required.

Ex. To find the log. sine of 1° 52' 54'' 25''' or 1° 52' 54'' $\frac{25}{60}$ or $\frac{5}{12}$.

Here the sine of 1° 52' 54'' taken from the next leaves 641, which multiplied by 5 and divided by 12, or multiplied by 25 and divided by 60, gives 267 the pro. part; this added to the first sine gives that which was required.

1° 52' 54'' sine	8·5163420
1 52 55 -	8·5164061
	dif. 641
	5
	12)3205
pro. part.	267
1° 52' 54'' -	8·5163420
1° 52' 54'' 25'''	8·5163687

On the contrary, if a sine or tangent be given, to find the corresponding arc; take the difference between it and the next less tabular number, and the difference between the next less and greater tabular numbers, so shall the less difference be the numerator, and the greater the denominator, of the fractional part to be added to the arc of the less tabular number; which fraction may also, if required, be either turned into a decimal, or into 3ds &c, by multiplying the numerator by 60, and dividing by the denominator.

Ex. To find the arc whose sine is 8·5163900.

Finding the number is between the sines of 1° 52' 55'' and 1° 52' 54'', take the differences between the sines as in the margin, and the differences give $\frac{480}{641}$ for the fraction of a second, or $\frac{48}{64}$ nearly, which abbreviates to $\frac{3}{4}'' = 45'''$; and therefore the arc sought is 1° 52' 54'' 45'''.

1° 52' 55'' -	8·5164061
1 52 54	8·5163420
1 52 54 45'''	8·5163900
diff. - -	480
diff. - -	641

Where the 1st differences of the sines and tangents alter much, as near the beginning of the table, the 2d, 3d, &c, differences may be taken in, and then the logarithmic sine or tangent will be expressed by this series, viz.

$$Q = A + x D' + x.\frac{x-1}{2}D'' + x.\frac{x-1}{2}.\frac{x-2}{3}D''' \text{ &c, or nearly } A + \overline{D' - \tfrac{1}{2}D''}.x;$$

where A is the next less tabular logarithm, D', D'', D''', &c, the 1st, 2d, 3d, &c, differences of the tabular logarithms, and x the fractional part of the arc over the complete seconds.

Ex. To find the log. tangent of 5′ 1″ 12‴ 24⁗ or 5′ 1″ $\frac{64}{300}$ or 5′ 1″ ·206.

Tang.		D′		Here A = 7·1641417; $x = \frac{62}{300}$; D′ = 14404;
5′ 0″	- 7·1626964	14453	D″	and the mean 2d diff. D″ = −48. Hence
5 1	- 7·1641417	14404	-49	A - - - 7·1641417
5 2	- 7·1655821	14357	-47	x D′ - - - - 2977
5 3	- 7·1670178			$x . \dfrac{x-1}{2}$D″ - - - - 4

Therefore the tangent of 5′ 1″ 12‴ 24⁗ - - - - $\overline{7·1644398}$

And on the other hand, when the sine or tangent is given, and falls near the beginning of the table, from the same series we may find x the fractional part of a second. For suppose it be required to find the arc whose tangent is 7·1644398. This falling between the tangents of 5′ 1″ and 5′ 2″, take the differences, &c, as above, and the series gives $7·1644398 = 7·1641417 + x$ D′ $+ x . \dfrac{x-1}{2}$D″;

or $2981 = 14404\, x - 24 . \overline{x^2 - x}$, or $- 24\, x^2 + 14428\, x = 2981$; which gives $x = ·2067″$ nearly $= 12‴\ 24⁗$. Therefore the arc required is 5′ 1″ 12‴ 24⁗. Or rather the approximate value A + D′ $- \frac12$D″ $. x =$ Q, gives $x = \dfrac{Q - A}{D' - \frac12 D''} = \dfrac{2981}{14404 + 24} = \dfrac{2981}{14428} = ·2067$, the same as before.

OF THE LARGE TABLE OF NATURAL AND LOGARITH-MIC SINES, TANGENTS, SECANTS, AND VERSED SINES.

Table 10, page 248 - - - - 337, contains all the sines, tangents, secants, and versed sines, both natural and logarithmic, to every minute of the quadrant, the degrees at top, and minutes descending down the left-hand side as far as 45°, or the middle of the quadrant, and from thence returning with the degrees at the bottom, and the minutes ascending by the right-hand side to 90°, or the other half of the quadrant, in such sort, that any arc on the one side is on the same line with its complement on the other side; the respective sines, cosines, tangents, cotangents, &c, being on the same line with the minutes, and in the columns signed with their respective names, at top when the degrees are at top, but at the bottom when the degrees are at the bottom. The natural sines, tangents, &c, are placed all together on the left-hand pages, and the logarithmic ones all together, facing them, on the right-hand pages. Also in the naturals there are two columns of the common differences, and in the logarithmic 3 columns of common differences, each column of differences being placed between the two columns of numbers having the same differences; so that these differences serve for both their right-hand and left-hand adjacent columns: also each differential number is set opposite the space between the numbers whose difference it is. The numbers on the same line in those columns having such common differences, are mutually complements of each other; so that the sum of the decimal figures of any two such numbers, is always 1 integer, with 0 in each place of decimals.

All this will be evident by inspecting one page of each sort, as well as the method of taking out the sine, &c, to any degrees and complete minutes. It is however to be observed, that in all the log. sines, tangents, &c, and in such of the natural as have any significant figure for their index or characteristic, the indices are expressed in the table, and the separating point is placed between the index and the decimal part of the number; but in several columns of the natural sines, &c, having 0 for their integer or index, both the index and decimal separating point are omitted; and whereever this is the case, it is to be understood that all the figures in such columns are decimals, wanting before them only the separating point and index 0.

The sine, tangent, or secant of any arc, has the same value, or is expressed by the same number, as the sine, tangent, or secant of the supplement of that arc; for which reason the tables are carried only to a quadrant or 90 degrees. So that when an arc is greater than 90^0, subtract it from 180^0, and take the sine, tang. or secant of the remainder, for that of the arc given. But this property does not take place between the versed sines of arcs and their supplements: and to find the versed sine of an arc greater than 90^0, proceed thus: in the natural versed sines, to radius add the natural cosine, the sum will be the natural versed sine; and in the log. versed sines, add 0·3010300 to twice the log. sine of half the arc, the sum, abating radius 10·0000000, will be the log. versed sine required.

1. *Given any Arc; to find its Sine, Cosine, Tangent, &c.*

Seek the degrees at the top or bottom, and the minutes respectively on the left or right; then on the same line with these is the sine, &c, each in its proper column, the title being at the top or bottom, according as the degrees are.

But when the given arc contains any parts of a minute, intermediate to those found in the table: take the difference between the tabular sines, &c, of the given degrees and minutes, and of the minute next greater; then take the proportional part of that difference for the parts of the minute, and add to it the sine, tangent, secant, and versed sine, or subtract it from the cosine, cotangent, cosecant, or coversed sine, of the given degrees and minutes; so shall the sum or remainder be the sine, &c, required.

Note, The proportional part is found thus, as $1'$ is to the given intermediate part of a minute, so is the whole difference to the proportional part required; which therefore is found by multiplying the difference by the said intermediate part. Also that intermediate part may be expressed either by a vulgar fraction, or a decimal, or a sexagesimal in seconds, thirds, &c, and the fraction or sexagesimal may be first reduced to a decimal, if it be thought better so to do, by dividing the numerator of the fraction by the denominator, or by dividing the sexagesimal by 60.

EXAMPLES.

1. To find the natural sine of
1° 48′ 28″ 12‴.

In the column of difference between the natural sines of 1° 48′ and 1° 49′ is the difference 2907 ; and 28″ 12‴ being = 28·2″ = ·47′; therefore as 1 : 2907 : : ·47 : the pro. part +1306
to which add sin. 1° 48′   0314168
makes sin. of 1° 48′ 28″ 12‴ $\overline{0315474}$

2. To find the natural tangent of
8° 9′ 10″ 24‴

8° 10′ tang. - -	1435084
8 9 - -	1432115
	diff. 2969

1 : 2969 : : (10″ 24‴ =) ·17′¼: + 515
   8° 9′ - -   1432115
   8° 9′ 10″ 24‴ - $\overline{1432630}$

3. To find the nat. coversed sine of
4° 6′ 5″ 40‴.

1 : 2902 (tab. dif.) : : $\frac{17}{180}$′ = } −274
   5″ 40‴: pro. part - }
   4° 6′ covers - - 9285026
   4° 6′ 5″ 40‴ - $\overline{9284752}$

4. To find the logarithmic cosine of
6° 8′ 42″

1:136(tab.dif.):::7′=42″: pr. pt. - 95
   6° 8′ cosine -   9·9975069
   6° 8′ 42″ - - $\overline{9·9974974}$

5. To find the log. sec. of 7° 12′ 50″.
1:160tab.dif.::⅚′=50″: pr. pt.+133
   7° 12′ secant - 10·0034381
   7° 12′ 50″ - $\overline{10·0034514}$

6. To find the logarithm cotangent of
39° 4′ 12′ 20‴.

1 : 2581 tab. dif. : : ·20⅝ = } −531
   12″ 20‴: pro. part. }
   39° 4′ cotan. - 10·0905978
   39° 4′ 12″ 20‴ - $\overline{10·0905447}$

The foregoing method of finding the proportional part of the tabular difference, to be added or subtracted, by one single proportion, is only true when those differences are nearly equal, and may do for all except for the tangents and secants of large arcs near the end of the quadrant in the natural sines, &c, and in the log. sines, &c, except the sines and versed sines of small arcs, the tangents of both large and small arcs, and the secants of large arcs. And when much accuracy is required, these excepted parts may be found by the series used in the last article, viz. $Q = A + x D' + x . \frac{x-1}{2} D'' + x . \frac{x-1}{2} . \frac{x-2}{3} D'''$ &c. or $= A + \overline{D' - \frac{1}{2}D''} . x$ nearly; where A is the tabular number for the degrees and minutes, D', D'', D''', &c, the 1st, 2d, 3d, &c tabular differences, and x the fractional part over the complete minutes, &c; at least it may be proper to find the tangents and secants of very large arcs from this series; but as to the log. sines, versed sines, and tangents of small arcs, they may also be found, perhaps easier, from their corresponding natural ones, viz. find the natural sine, versed sine, or tangent of the given small arc, and then find the log. of such natural number by the 1st or large table of logarithms, which will be the log. sine, &c, required. And the log. tangent and secant of large arcs will be also found by taking the difference between 20 and their log. cotangent and cosine respectively. And lastly, the natural tangents and secants of large arcs may also be found by first finding their log. tangent and secant, and then finding the corresponding number.

EXAMPLES.

1. To find the log. sine of 1° 48′ 28″ 12‴.
The natural sine, found in Ex. 1. above is ·0315474; and the log. of this is 8·4989636 which is the log. sine required.

2. To find the log. vers. of 1° 48′ 28″ 12‴
$$1° 48′ \text{ nat. vers.} \quad - - - \quad 0004934$$
$$1 : 92 \text{ tab. dif.} : : ·47′ = 28″ 12‴ : + 43$$
$$1° 48′ 28″ 12‴ \text{ nat. vers.} \quad - ·0004977$$
Its log. 1 48 28 12 log. vers.   6·6969676

3. To find the log. tang. of 2° 23′ 33″ 36‴.
$$2° 23′ \text{ its nat. tan.} \quad - - \quad 0416210$$
$$1 : 2914 \text{ tab. dif.} : : : ·56′ = 33″ 36‴ : + 1632$$
$$2° 23′ 33″ 36‴ \text{ nat. tan.} \quad - \quad 0417842$$
Its log. 2 23 33 36 log. tang.   8·6210121

4. To find the log. tang. of 87° 36′ 26″ 24‴.
Its complement is - - - 2 23 33 36
Whose log. tang. in Ex. 3 is   8·6210121
Taken from - - - - - 20·0000000
Leaves log. tan. 87° 36′ 26″ 24‴ 11·3789879

5. To find the log. sec. of 88° 11′ 31″ 48‴.
Its complement is - - 1 48 28 12
Its log. sine in Ex. 1 is - - 8·4989636
Which taken from - - - 20·0000000
Leaves lo. sec. 88° 11′ 31″ 48‴ L1·5010364

6. To find the nat. sec. of 88° 11′ 31″ 48‴.

	nat. sec.	D′	D″	D‴
88° 9′	30·976074	281503		
88 10	31·257577	286669	5166	
88 11	31·544246	291979	5310	144
88 12	31·836225	297438	5459	149
88 13	32·133663			

Hence A = 31·544246; D′ = 291979;
D″ = 5310; the mean D‴ = 146;
$$x = ·53′ = 31″ 48‴; \quad x . \frac{x-1}{2} = -·12455;$$
$$x . \frac{x-1}{2} . \frac{x-2}{3} = ·06125,$$

Then A - - - - - - - 31·544246
$$x \, D′ \quad - - - - - - - \quad 154748$$
$$x . \frac{x-1}{2} D″ \quad - - - - - \quad -664$$
$$x . \frac{x-1}{2} . \frac{x-2}{3} D‴ \quad - - - - - \quad 9$$
               31·698339

In the 6th example, the natural secant is found by the differential series to be 31·698339. But by taking the number to the logarithm of it, as found in the 5th example, it is 31·698333; which seems to be the more accurate, as well as the easier way; and indeed this method by the series seems to be, in some instances, more troublesome, and less accurate, than finding the secant by dividing 1 by the cosine.

2. *Given any Sine, Tangent, &c. to find its Arc.*

Take the difference between the next less and greater tabular numbers of the same kind, and the difference between the given number
and said next less or next greater tabular number, according as the
given number is a sine, tangent, &c, or a cosine, cotangent, &c, noting
its degrees and minutes ; then the two differences will be the terms of
a vulgar fraction of a minute, to be added to those minutes, to give the
arc required.

And this vulgar fraction may also, if required, be reduced to a decimal by dividing the less or numerator by the denominator, or brought
to sexigesimals, by multiplying by 60, &c. Also, where the tabular
differences are printed, the subtraction of the less tabular number from
the greater is saved.

EXAMPLES.

1. To find the arc to the natural sine
             ·0315474.
Ans. 1° 48′ 28″ 12‴ 0315474
Subtr. 1 48′ next less 0314108
                       ————
                        1366
                          60
                       ————
Tab. diff. - 2907) 81960 (28″
                      5814
                      ————
                      23820
                      23256
                      ————
                        564
                         60
                      ————
            2907) 33840 (12‴

2. To find the arc to natural tang.
             ·1432630
Next greater   -   1435084
Ans. 8° 9′ 10″ 24‴ 1432630
Next less,subt. fr. each 1432115
                         ————
                          515
                           60
                         ————
Tab. difference 2969) 30900 (10″
                        29690
                        ————
                         1210
                           60
                        ————
                        72600 (24‴
                        5938
                        ————
                       13220

3. To find the arc to logarithm cosine
             9·9974974.
        6° 8′   -   9·9975069
Answer 6° 8′ 42″ 9·9974974
                   ————
                     95
                     60
                   ————
Tab. difference   136)5700
                      544
                      ————
                      260

4. To find the arc to logarithm cot.
             10·0905447.
        39° 4′   -   10.0905978
Ans. 39° 4′ 12″ 20‴ 10·0905447
                     ————
                      531
                       60
                     ————
Tab. difference 2581) 31860 (12″
                       2581
                       ————
                       6050
                       5162
                       ————
                        888
                         60
                       ————
                2581) 53280 (20‴
                       5162
                       ————
                       1660

The above method of proportioning by the first difference alone, can only be true when the other differences are nothing, or very small; but other means must be used when they are large, viz. for the natural tangents and secants of very large arcs; and for the logarithmic sines, and versed sines of small arcs, also the log. secants of large arcs, with the log. tangents and cotangents both of small and large arcs. When the log. sine, versed sine, or tangent of a small arc is given, by means of the table of logarithms find the corresponding natural number, and then the arc answering to it in the table of natural sines, &c. But when the log. tangent or secant of a large arc is proposed, subtract it from 20, the remainder is the log. cotangent or cosine, which will be the log. tangent or sine of a small arc which is the complement of that required, which complement will be found as in the last remark, by taking the corresponding natural number, and finding it in the natural tangents or sines; then subtracting that complemental arc from 90°, leaves the required large arc answering to the proposed log. tangent or secant. And when the natural tangent or secant of a large arc is proposed, change it into the log. tangent or secant of the same, by taking the log. of the proposed natural number; then proceed with it as above in the last remark.—Or, what relates to the log. sines and tangents of small arcs, or cosines and cotangents of large ones, will be best performed by the foregoing table for every second of the first 2 degrees.

EXAMPLES.

1. To find the arc to natural tangent 50·0000000.

$$20·0000000$$

Given 50·0000000 its log. 11·6989700

·02 - - - - 8·3010300

·0197830 nat. tan. of 1° 8'

2170
60

2910) 130200 (44"
1164

1380
1164

216
60

12960 (44'''
1164

1320

Hence from - -	90°	0' 0" 0'''
Take the comp. -	1	8 44 44
Leaves arc required	88	51 15 16

2. To find the arc to natural secant 31·6983333.

$$20·0000000$$

Given 31·698⅓ its log. 11·5010365

·0315474 - - 8·4989635

·0314108 nat. sine of 1° 48'

1366
60

2907) 81960 (28"
5814

23820
23256

564
60

33840 (12'''
2907

4770

Hence from -	90°	0' 0" 0''
Take the comp.	1	48 28 12
Leaves arc required	88	11 31 48

X 2

TRIGONOMETRICAL RULES,

1. **I**N a right-lined triangle, whose sides are A, B, C, and their opposite angles, a, b, c; having given any three of these, of which one is a side; to find the rest.

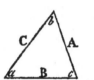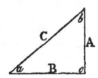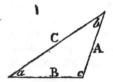

Put s for the sine, s' the cosine, t the tangent, and t' the cotangent, of an arch or angle, to the radius r; also L for a logarithm, and L′ its arithmetical complement. Then

Case 1. When three sides A, B, C, are given.

Put $\mathrm{P} = \frac{1}{2}.\ \overline{\mathrm{A} + \mathrm{B} + \mathrm{C}}$ or semiperimeter.

Then $s.\ \frac{1}{2}\,c = r\sqrt{\dfrac{(\mathrm{P}-\mathrm{A})\times(\mathrm{P}-\mathrm{B})}{\mathrm{A}\times\mathrm{B}}}$.

And $s'.\ \frac{1}{2}\,c = r\sqrt{\dfrac{\mathrm{P}\times(\mathrm{P}-\mathrm{C})}{\mathrm{A}\times\mathrm{B}}}$.

L. $s.\frac{1}{2}c = \frac{1}{2}.\ (\mathrm{L.}\ \overline{\mathrm{P}-\mathrm{A}} + \mathrm{L.}\ \overline{\mathrm{P}-\mathrm{B}} + \mathrm{L}'\,\mathrm{A} + \mathrm{L}'\,\mathrm{B})$.
L′ $s.\frac{1}{2}c = \frac{1}{2}\ (\mathrm{L.}\ \mathrm{P} + \mathrm{L.}\ \overline{\mathrm{P}-\mathrm{C}} + \mathrm{L}'\,\mathrm{A} + \mathrm{L}'\,\mathrm{B})$.

Note, When A = B, then

$s.\ \frac{1}{2}c = \dfrac{c}{\mathrm{A}} \times \dfrac{r}{2}$. And $s'\ \frac{1}{2}c = r\sqrt{\dfrac{\mathrm{A}^2 - \frac{1}{4}\,\mathrm{c}^2}{\mathrm{A}^2}}$.

Case 2. Given two sides A, B, and their included angle c.

Put $s = 90° - \frac{1}{2}c$, and $t.\ d = \dfrac{\mathrm{A}-\mathrm{B}}{\mathrm{A}+\mathrm{B}} \times t.\ s$; then $a = s + d$; and $b = s - d$. And

$c = \sqrt{\left(\dfrac{4\mathrm{A}\,\mathrm{B}\times \mathrm{s}^2\frac{1}{2}c}{rr} + \overline{\mathrm{A}-\mathrm{B}}\big)^2\right)}$.

Or in logarithms, putting L. Q = 2L. $(\mathrm{A}-\mathrm{B})$. and L. R = L. 2A + L. 2B + 2L. s. $\frac{1}{2}$ $c-20$,
then L. C = $\frac{1}{2}$ L. (Q+R).

If the angle c be right, or = 90°; then

$t.\ a = \dfrac{\mathrm{A}}{\mathrm{B}}\,r$; $t.\ b = \dfrac{\mathrm{B}}{\mathrm{A}}\,r$;

$c = \dfrac{r}{s.a}\mathrm{A}$, or $= \dfrac{r}{s.b}\mathrm{B}$, or $= \sqrt{\mathrm{A}^2+\mathrm{B}^2}$.

If A = B; then
$a = b = 90° - \frac{1}{2}c$, and $\left.\right\}\ c = \dfrac{s.\frac{1}{2}c}{r}\times 2\mathrm{A}$.

Case 3. When a side and its opposite angle are among the terms given.

Then $\dfrac{\mathrm{A}}{s.a} = \dfrac{\mathrm{B}}{s.b} = \dfrac{\mathrm{C}}{s.c}$; from which equations any term wanted may be found.

When an angle, as a, is 90°, and A and c are given, then

B $= \sqrt{(\mathrm{A}^2-\mathrm{C}^2)} = \sqrt{(\mathrm{A}+\mathrm{C})\times(\mathrm{A}-\mathrm{C})}$.
And L. B $= \frac{1}{2}$ (L. $\overline{\mathrm{A}+\mathrm{C}}$ + L. $\overline{\mathrm{A}-\mathrm{C}}$).

Note, When two sides A, B, and an angle a opposite to one of them, are given; if A be less than B, then b, c, c, have each two values; otherwise, only one value.

II. In a spheric triangle, whose three sides are A, B, C, and their opposite angles, a, b, c; any three of these six terms being given, to find the rest.

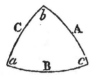 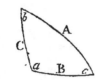

Case 1. Given the three sides A, B, C. Calling 2P the perim. or P $= \frac{1}{2}$(A+B+C).

Then s. $\frac{1}{2}c = r\sqrt{\dfrac{\text{s. (P}-\text{A)} \times \text{s. (P}-\text{B)}}{\text{s. A} \times \text{s. B}}}$.

And s'$\frac{1}{2}c = r\sqrt{\dfrac{\text{s. P} \times \text{s. (P}-c)}{\text{s. A} \times \text{s. B}}}$.

L. s.$\frac{1}{2}c = \frac{1}{2}$(L. s. $\overline{\text{P}-\text{A}}$ + L. s. $\overline{\text{P}-\text{B}}$ + L's. A + L's. B)

L. s'$c = \frac{1}{2}$(L. s. P + L. s. $\overline{\text{P}-\text{C}}$ + L' s. A + L' s. B).

And the same for the other angles.

Case 2. Given the three angles.

Put $2p = a + b + c$. Then

s $\frac{1}{2}c = r\sqrt{\dfrac{\text{s'}p \times \text{s'}(p-c)}{\text{s. }a \times \text{s. }b}}$. And

s'$\frac{1}{2}c = r\sqrt{\dfrac{\text{s'}(p-a) \times \text{s'}(p-b)}{\text{s. }a \times \text{s. }b}}$.

L. s. $\frac{1}{2}c = \frac{1}{2}$(L. s'$p$ + L. s' $\overline{p-c}$ + L' s. a + L' s. b)

L. s'$\frac{1}{2}c = \frac{1}{2}$(L. s' $\overline{p-a}$ + L. s' $\overline{p-b}$ + L' s. a + L' s. b)

And the same for the other sides.

Note, The sign 7 signifies greater than, and ∠ less than; also ∽ the difference.

Case 3. Given A, B, and included angle c.

To find an angle a opposite the side A, let $r : s'c :: t.$ A $: t.$ M, like or unlike A, as c is 7 or ∠ 90°; also N $=$ B ∽ M:

then s. N $:$ s. M $::$ t. $c :$ t. a, like or unlike c as M is 7 or ∠ B.

Or let s' $\frac{1}{2}$. A $+$ B $:$ s'.$\frac{1}{2}$. A ∽ B $:: t'$ $\frac{1}{2}c :$ t. M, which is 7 or ∠ 90°. as A $+$ B is 7 or ∠ 180°. and s.$\frac{1}{2}$. A $+$ B $:$ s. A ∽ B $:: t'$ $\frac{1}{2}c: t.$ N, 7 90°, then $a =$ M $+$ N; and $b =$ M $-$ N.

Again let $r : s'c :: t.$ A $: t.$ M, like or unlike A as c is 7 or ∠ 90°; and N $=$ B ∽ M.

Then s' M $:$ s' N $::$ s'A $:$ s' c, like or unlike N as c is 7 or ∠ 90°. Or,

s. $\frac{1}{2}$ c $= \sqrt{\dfrac{\text{s. A} \times \text{s. B} \times \text{s}^2 \frac{1}{2}c}{rr} + \text{s}^2\frac{1}{2}.\text{A} ∽ \text{B}}$.

In logarithms, put L. Q $=$ 2 L. s. $\frac{1}{2}$ A ∽ B; and L. R $=$ L. s. A $+$ L. s. B $+$ 2 L. s. $\frac{1}{2}c - 20$; then L. s. $\frac{1}{2}$ c $= \frac{1}{2}$ L. (Q $+$ R).

Case 4. Given a, b, and included side C.

First, let $r : s'$ c $:: t.$ $a : t'$ m, like or unlike a as c is 7 or ∠ 90°; also $n = b$ ∽ m. Then s' $n :$ s' $m :: t.$ c $: t.$ A, like or unlike n as a is 7 or ∠ 90°.

Or, let s' $\frac{1}{2}.\overline{a + b} :$ s'$\frac{1}{2}. a$ ∽ $b :: t.\frac{1}{2}$ c $: t.$ M, 7 or ∠ 90° as $a + b$ is 7 or ∠ 180°; and s. $\frac{1}{2}\overline{a + b} :$ s.$\frac{1}{2}a$∽$b :: t.\frac{1}{2}$ c $: t.$ N, 7 90°; then A $=$ M $\pm$ N; and B $=$ M $\mp$ N.

Again, let $r : s'$ c $:: t.$ $a : t'$ m, like or unlike a as c is 7 or ∠ 90°; and $n = b$ ∽ m:

then s. $m.$ $:$ s. $n :: s'$ $a : s'$ c, like or unlike a as m is 7 or ∠ b.

Case 5. Given A, B, and an opposite angle a.

1st. s. A $:$ s. $a :: $ s. B $:$ s. b, 7 or ∠ 90°.

2nd. Let $r : s'$B $:: t.$ $a : t'$ m, like or unlike B as a is 7 or ∠ 90°; and t. A $: t.$ B $:: s'$ $m : s'$ n, like or unlike A as a is 7 or ∠ 90°; then $c = m \pm n$, two values also.

3dly. Let $r : s'$ $a :: t.$ B $: t.$ M, like or unlike B as a is 7 or ∠ 90°; and s' B $:$ s'A $:: s'$M $: s'$ N, like or unlike A as a is 7 or ∠ 90°; then C $=$ M $\pm$ N, two values also.

But if A be equal to B, or to its supplement, or between B and its supplement; then is b like to B: also c is $= m \pm n$, and $c =$ M $\mp$ N, as B is like or unlike a.

Case 6. Given *a*, *b*, and an opposite side A.

1st. s. *a* : s. A. : : s. *b* : s. B, 〉 or ∠ 90°.

2nd. Let *r* : s′ *b* : : t. A : t. M, like or unlike
　　　b as A is 〉 or ∠ 90°;
and t. *a* : t. *b* : : s. M. : s. N, 〉 or ∠ 90° :
then c = M ± N, as *a* is like or unlike *b*.

3dly. Let *r* : s′ A : : t. *b* : t′ m, like or un-
　　　like *b* as A 〉 or ∠ 90°;
and s′ *b* : s′ *a* : : s. m : s. n, 〉 or ∠ 90° :
then c = m ± n, as *a* is like or unlike *b*.

But if A be equal to B, or to its supplement, or between B and its supplement;
then B is unlike *b*, and only the less values
of N, *n*, are possible.

Note, When two sides A, B, and their opposite angles *a*, *b*, are known; the third
side c, and its opposite angle c, are readily
found thus:

s. ½ *a* ꝏ *b* : s. ½. *a* + *b* : : t. ½ A ꝏ B : t. ½ c.
s. ½. A ꝏ B : s. ½. A + B : : t. ½. *a* ꝏ *b* : t. ½ c.

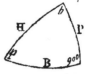 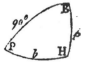

III. In a right-angled spheric triangle,
where H is the hypotenuse, or side opposite
the right angle, B, P, the other two sides, and
b, *p*, their opposite angles; any two of these
five terms being given, to find the rest; the
cases, with their solutions, are as in the following table.

The same table will also serve for the
quadrantal triangle, or that which has one
side = 90°, H being the angle opposite to
that side, B, P, the other two angles, and *b*,
p, their opposite sides: observing, instead of
H to take its supplement: or else mutually
changing the terms *like* and *unlike* for each
other where H is concerned, and its real
value is taken.

Case	Given	Req^d	SOLUTIONS.
1	H B	b p P	s. H : *r* : : s.B : s.*b*, and is like B *r* : t′.H : : t.B : s′.*p* } 〉 or ∠ 90° as H is like or unlike B s′. B : *r* : : s′.H : s.P
2	H b	B P p	*r* : s.H : : s.*b* : s.B, like *b* *r* : s′.*b* : : t.H : t.P } 〉 or ∠ 90° as H is like or unlike *b* *r* : s′.H : : t.*b* : t′.*p*
3	B b	H P p	s.*b* : *r* : : s.B : s.H } *r* : t.B : : t′.*b* : s.P } , each 〉 or ∠ 90°; both values true s′.B : *r* : : s.*b* : s.*p*
4	B p	H b P	*r* : t′.B : : s′.*p* : t′.H, 〉 or ∠ 90° as B is like or unlike *p* *r* : s′.B : : s.*p* : s′.*b*, like B *r* : s.B : : t.*p* : t.P, like *p*
5	B p	H b p	*r* : s′.B : : s′.P : s′.H, ∠ or 〉 90° as B is like or unlike P *r* : s.P : : t′.B : t′.*b*, like B *r* : s.B : : t.P : t.*p*, like P
6	p b	H B P	*r* : t′.*b* : : t′.*p* : s′.H, 〉 or ∠ 90° as *b* is like or unlike *p* s.*p* : *r* : : s′.*b* : s′.B, like *b* s.*b* : *r* : : s′.*p* : s′.P, like *p*

The following Propositions and Remarks, concerning Spherical Triangles, (selected and communicated by the Reverend Nevil Maskelyne, D. D. Astronomer Royal, F. R. S.) will also render the Calculation of them perspicuous, and free from Ambiguity.

" 1. A spherical triangle is equilateral, isoscelar, or scalene, according as it has its three angles all equal, or two of them equal, or all three unequal; and *vice versa*.

2. The greatest side is always opposite the greatest angle, and the smallest side opposite the smallest angle.

3. Any two sides taken together, are greater than the third.

4. If the three angles are all acute, or all right, or all obtuse; the three sides will be, accordingly, all less than 90°, or equal to 90°, or greater than 90°; and *vice versa*.

5. If from the three angles A, B, C, of a triangle ABC, as poles, there be described, upon the surface

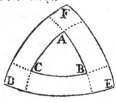

of the sphere, three arches of a great circle DE, DF, FE, forming by their intersections a new spherical triangle DEF; each side of the new triangle will be the supplement of the angle at its pole; and each angle of the same triangle, will be the supplement of the side opposite to it in the triangle A B C.

6. In any triangle A B C, or A *b* C, right angled in A, 1st, The angles at the hypotenuse are always of the same kind

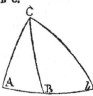

as their opposite sides; 2dly, The hypotenuse is less or greater than a quadrant according as the sides including the right angle are of the same or different kinds; that is to say, according as these same sides are either both acute or both obtuse, or as one is acute and the other obtuse. And, *vice versa*, 1st, The sides including the right angle, are always of the same kind as their opposite angles: 2dly, The sides including the right angle will be of the same or different kinds, according as the hypotenuse is less or more than 90°: but one at least of them will be of 90°, if the hypotenuse is so."

THE CASES OF PLANE TRIANGLES RESOLVED BY LOGARITHMS.

IN this and the following solutions of spherical triangles, it is to be observed, that when we say the sine, tangent, &c, we mean the logarithmic sine, tangent, &c, as found by the table.

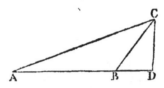

Prop. I. *Having the angles, and one side; to find either of the other sides.*

Add the logarithm of the given side to the sine of the angle opposite to the side required, and from the sum subtract the sine of the angle opposed to the given side; the remainder will be the logarithm of the side required.

Example. In the triangle BCD, having the angle CDB 90°, CBD 51° 56′, BCD 38° 4′ and the side BD 197·3 ; to find the side CD.

2·2951271 log. of 197·3.
9·8961369 sin. of 51° 56′
───────────
12·1912640 sum
9·7899880 sin. of 38·4
───────────
2·4012760 log. 251·9278 CD req.

Or you may add the complement of the sine of the angle opposed to the given side, to the two other logarithms, the sum (abating radius) is the logarithm of the side required ; as shown in art. 3 of Log. Arith. And it is to be observed that the complements of the sines in the table are to be found in the columns of the cosecants : for (passing over the first

unit) the cosecants of the same arcs are the complements of the same sines. Also the complements of the tangents, are the cotangents.

Example. The sine of 38° 4′ being 9·7899880, the cosecant of 38° 4′ is 10·2100120,which (omitting the first unit) is the complement of the said sine.

0·2100120 co. of sin. 38° 4′
2·2951271 log. of 197·3
9·8961369 sin. of 51° 56′
───────────
2·4012760 log. 251·9278, as before.

But if one side and the angles, of a right-angled triangle, be known, and you would have the other side, as in the former example, the operation will be easier thus :

Add the tangent of the angle opposite to the side required, to the logarithm of the given side, the sum (abating radius) is the logarithm of the side required.

10·1061489 tan. 51° 56′
2·2951271 log. of 197·3
───────────
2·4012760 log. 251·9278 as before.

Prop. II. *Having two sides, and an angle opposite to one of them ; to find the other two angles, and the third side.*

Add the sine of the angle given, to the logarithm of the side adjoining that angle, and from the sum subtract the logarithm of the side opposite to that angle, or add its arithmetical comp. the remainder or sum will be the sine of the angle opposite to the adjoining side.

Example. In the triangle A B C, having the side AC 800, BC 320, and the angle ABC 128° 4'; to find the angles BAC, ACB, and the side AB.

7·0969100 ar. com. log. 800.
2·5051500 log. of 320.
9·8961369 sin. 128° 4'.
0·4981969 sin.   18 21 BAC.

Having BAC and ABC, the angle ACB is their supplement to 180°, viz. 33° 35'; and you may find the side AB by the first proposition.

Prop. III. *Having two sides and the angle between them; to find the other two angles, and the third side.*

If the angle included be a right angle, add the radius to the logarithm of the less side, and from the sum subtract the logarithm of the greater side, or add its arith. comp.: the remainder or sum will be the tangent of the angle opposed to the less side.

· *Example.* In the triangle BCD, having the side BE 197·3, and CD 251·9; to find the angles BCD, CBD, and the side CB.

7·5987728 ar. com. log. 251·9
12·2951271 rad. + log. 197·3
9·8938989 tan. 38° 4' BCD.

But if the angle included be oblique, add the logarithm of the difference of the given sides to the tangent of half the sum of the unknown angles, and from the sum subtract the logarithm of the sum of the given sides, or add its complement; the remainder or sum will be the tangent of half their difference.

· *Example.* In the triangle ABC, having the side AB 562, BC 320, and the angle ABC 128° 4'; to find the angles BAC, ACB, and the side AC.

The sum of the given sides is 882, and the difference 242, the half sum of the unknown angles is 25₀ 58'.

7·0545314 com. log. 882
2·3838154 log. of 242
9·6875402 tang. 25° 58'
9·1258870 tang. 7 37
                    25 58
Angle ACB - 33 35 sum,
Angle CAB - 18 21 dif.

These 7° 37' being added to 25° 58' the half-sum of the angles unknown, the sum is 33° 35' for the greater angle ACB; and the same 7° 37' being subtracted from 25° 58', the remainder is 18° 21' for the lesser angle CAB. Lastly, knowing the angles, and two sides, the third side may be found by the first proposition.

Prop. IV. *Having the three sides; to find any angle.*

Add the three sides together, and take half the sum, and the differences betwixt the half-sum and each side: then add the complements of the logarithms of the half-sum, and of the difference between the half-sum and the side opposite to the angle sought; to the logarithms of the differences of the half-sum, and the other sides, half their sum will be the tangent of half the angle required.

Example. In the triangle A B C, having the side AB 562, AC 800, and BC 320; to find the angle ABC.

AC = 800	H=841	-	co. 7·0752040
AB = 562	H−AC=41	co·	8·3872161
BC = 320	H−AB=279	-	2·4956042
sum 1682	H−BC=521	-	2·7168377
½ sum 841 =H		sum	20·6248620

Tang. of 64°2'=½ sum 10·3124310
Whose double 128° 4' is the angle ABC.

THE CASES OF SPHERICAL TRIANGLES RESOLVED BY LOGARITHMS.

THE resolution of spherical triangles is to be performed by the table of sines, tangents, and secants; which we shall show by the 28 propositions following; whereof 16 are of right-angled, and 12 are of oblique triangles; and first

Of right-angled Triangles.

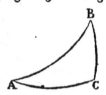

Prop. I. *Having the legs; to find the hypotenuse.*

Add the cosine of one leg, to the cosine of the other leg; the sum (abating radius) is the cosine of the hypotenuse required.

Example. In the right-angled triangle ABC, having AC 27° 54', and BC 11° 30'; to find AB the hypotenuse.

```
9·9911927 cosin. 11° 30'
9·9463371 cosin. 27  54
9·9375298 cosin. 30 AB req.
```

Prop. II. *Having the two legs; to find either of the angles.*

Add the sine of the leg next the angle sought, to the cotangent of the other leg: the sum (abating radius) is the cotangent of the angle required.

Example. In the right-angled triangle ABC, having AC 27° 54', and BC 11° 30'; to find the angle BAC.

```
9·6701807 sin. next leg 27° 54'
10·6915374 cot. opp. leg 11  30
10·3617181   cotan. BAC 23  30
```

Prop. III. *Having the hypotenuse, and one of the angles; to find the other angle.*

Add the cosine of the hypotenuse to the tangent of the angle given; the sum (abating radius) is the cotangent of the angle required.

Example. In the right-angled triangle ABC, having the hypotenuse AB 30°, and the angle ABC 69° 22'; to find the angle BAC.

```
9·9375306 cosin. hyp. AB  30° 00'
10·4241896 tang. ABC   -  69  22
10·3617202 cotan. BAC  -  23  30
```

Prop. IV. *Having the hypotenuse, and one of the angles; to find the leg next the given angle.*

Add the tangent of the hypotenuse to the cosine of the angle given; the sum (abating radius) is the tangent of the leg required.

Example. In the right-angled triangle ABC, having the hypotenuse AB 30°, and the angle ABC 69° 22'; to find the leg BC.

```
9·7614393 tang. hyp. AB  30° 00'
9·5470188 cosin. ABC   -  69  22
9·3084581 tang. BC   - -  11  30
```

Prop. V. *Having the hypotenuse, and one of the angles; to find the leg opposed to the given angle.*

Add the sine of the hypotenuse to the sine of the angle given; the sum (abating radius) is the sine of the leg required.

Example. In the right-angled triangle ABC, having the hypotenuse AB 30°, and the angle BAC 23° 30'; to find the leg BC.

```
9·6989700 sin. hyp. AB  30° 00'
9·6006997 sin. BAC   -  23  30
9·2996697 sin. BC   -  11  30
```

Prop. VI. *Having one of the legs and the angle next it; to find the hypotenuse.*

Add the cotangent of the given leg, to the cosine of the given angle; the sum (abating radius) is the cotangent of the hypotenuse required.

Example. In the right-angled triangle ABC, having the leg AC 27° 54', and the angle BAC 23° 30'; to find the hypotenuse AB.

$$
\begin{array}{llll}
10\text{·}2761563 & \text{cot. } \text{AC} & - & 27° \ 54' \\
9\text{·}9623977 & \text{cos. } \text{BAC} & - & 23 \ 30 \\
\hline
10\text{·}2385540 & \text{cot. hyp. } \text{AB} & . & 30 \ 00
\end{array}
$$

Prop. VII. *Having one of the legs, and the angle next it; to find the other leg.*

Add the sine of the leg given to the tangent of the angle given; the sum (abating radius) is the tangent of the leg required.

Example. In the right-angled triangle ABC, having the leg AC 27° 54', and the angle BAC 23° 30'; to find the leg BC.

$$
\begin{array}{llll}
9\text{·}6701807 & \text{sin. } \text{AC} & 27° \ 54' \\
9\text{·}6383019 & \text{tan. } \text{BAC} & 23 \ 30 \\
\hline
9\text{·}3084826 & \text{tan. } \text{BC} & 11 \ 30
\end{array}
$$

Prop. VIII. *Having one of the legs, and the angle next to it; to find the other angle.*

Add the cosine of the given leg to the sine of the given angle; the sum (abating radius) is the cosine of the angle required.

Example. In the right-angled triangle ABC, having the leg BC 11° 30', and the angle ABC 69° 22'; to find the angle BAC.

$$
\begin{array}{llll}
9\text{·}9911927 & \text{cos. } \text{BC} & 11° \ 30' \\
9\text{·}9712084 & \text{sin. } \text{ABC} & 69 \ 22 \\
\hline
9\text{·}9624011 & \text{cos. } \text{BAC} & 23 \ 30
\end{array}
$$

Prop. IX. *Having one of the legs, and the angle opposed unto it; to find the hypotenuse.*

Add the radius to the sine of the given leg, and from the sum subtract the sine of the given angle, or add its cosecant; the remainder or sum is the sine of the hypotenuse required.

Example. In the right-angled triangle ABC, having the leg BC 11° 30', and the angle BAC 23° 30'; to find the hypotenuse AB.

$$
\begin{array}{llll}
9\text{·}2996553 & \text{sin. } \text{BC} & 11° \ 30' \\
0\text{·}3993003 & \text{cos. } \text{BAC} & 23 \ 30, \\
\hline
9\text{·}6989556 & \text{sin. } \text{AB} & 30 \ \text{reqd.}
\end{array}
$$

Prop. X. *Having one of the legs, and the angle opposed unto it; to find the other leg.*

Add the tangent of the given leg, to the cotangent of the given angle; the sum (abating radius) is the sine of the leg required.

Example. In the right-angled triangle ABC, having the leg BC 11° 30', and the angle BAC 23° 30'; to find the leg AC.

$$
\begin{array}{llll}
9\text{·}3084626 & \text{tang. } \text{BC} & 11° \ 30' \\
10\text{·}3616981 & \text{cot. } \text{BAC} & 23 \ 30 \\
\hline
9\text{·}6701607 & \text{sin. } \text{AC} & 27 \ 54
\end{array}
$$

Prop. XI. *Having one of the legs, and the angle opposed unto it; to find the other angle.*

Add the radius to the cosine of the given angle, and from the sum subtract the cosine of the given leg, or add the secant; the remainder or sum is the sine of the angle required.

Example. In the right-angled triangle ABC, having the leg BC 11° 30', and the angle BAC 23° 30'; to find the angle ABC.

$$
\begin{array}{llll}
9\text{·}9623977 & \text{cos. } \text{BAC} & 23° \ 30' \\
0\text{·}0088073 & \text{sec. } \text{BC} & 11 \ 30 \\
\hline
9\text{·}9712050 & \text{sin. } \text{ABC} & 69 \ 22
\end{array}
$$

Prop. XII. *Having one of the legs, and the hypotenuse; to find the angle next the given leg.*

Add the tangent of the given leg, to the cotangent of the hypotenuse, the sum (abating radius) is the cosine of the angle required.

Example. In the right-angled triangle ABC, having the leg AC 27° 54′, and the hypotenuse AB 30°; to find the angle BAC.

9·7238436 tan. AC 27° 54′
10·2385606 cot. AB 30   00
———————
9·9624042 cosi. BAC 23 30

Prop. XIII. *Having one of the legs, and the hypotenuse; to find the angle opposed to the given leg.*

Add the radius to the sine of the given leg, and from the sum subtract the sine of the hypotenuse, or add its cosecant; the remainder or sum will be the sine of the angle required.

Example. In the right-angled triangle ABC, having the leg BC 11° 30′, and the hypotenuse AB 30°; to find the angle BAC.

9·2996553 sin. leg BC   11° 30′
0·3010300 cosec. hyp. AB 30   00
———————
9·6006853 sine of BAC   23   30

Prop. XIV. *Having one of the legs, and the hypotenuse; to find the other leg.*

Add the radius to the cosine of the hypotenuse, and from the sum subtract the cosine of the given leg, or add its secant; the remainder or sum is the cosine of the leg required.

Example. In the right-angled triangle ABC, having the leg BC 11° 30′, and the hypotenuse AB 30°; to find the leg AC.

9·9375306 cosin. AB 30° 00′
0·0088073 sec.   BC 11   30
———————
9·9463379 cosin. AC 27   54

Prop. XV. *Having the angles; to find the hypotenuse.*

Add the cotangent of one oblique angle to the cotangent of the other oblique angle; the sum (abating radius) is the cosine of the hypotenuse required.

Example. In the right-angled triangle ABC, having the angle BAC

23° 30′, and the angle ABC 69° 22′; to find the hypotenuse AB.

0·3616981 cot. BAC 23° 30′
9·5758104 cot. ABC 69   22
———————
9·9375085 cos. hyp. AB 30 00

Prop. XVI. *Having the angles; to find either of the legs.*

Add the radius to the cosine of either oblique angle, and from the sum subtract the sine of the other oblique angle, or add its cosecant; the remainder or sum will be the cosine of the leg opposite to the angle whose cosine was taken.

Example. In the right-angled triangle ABC, having the angle BAC 23° 30′, and the angle ABC 69° 22′; to find the leg BC.

9·9623977 cosin. BAC 23° 30′
0·0287916 cosec. ABC 69   22
———————
9·9911893 cosin. BC 11   30

Of Oblique Triangles.

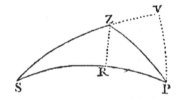

Prop. XVII. *Having the three sides, to find any of the angles.*

Add the three sides together, and take half the sum; also the difference between the half-sum and the side opposite to the angle sought. Then add the cosecants, or the complements of the sines, of the other sides, to the sines of the half-sum and of the said difference; half the sum of these four logarithms is the cosine of half the angle required.

Example. In the triangle SZP, having the side ZS 40°, PS 70°, and PZ 38° 30′; to find the angle ZPS.

PS = 70° 0′ cosec.   0·0270142
PZ = 38 30 cosec.   0·2058505
ZS = 40 0 sin. ½ sum 9·9833805
Sum 148 30 sin. dif. 9·7503579
¼ sum 74 15   2) 19·9666031
ZS = 40 0 cos. 15° 47′ 9·9833015
Diff. 34 15 ZPS 31 34 required.

Prop. XVIII. *Having the three angles ;*
to find any of the sides.

Let the angles be changed into sides, taking the supplement of one of them ; then the operation will be the same as in the former proposition.

Prop. XIX. *Having two angles, and a side opposed to one of them ; to find the side opposed to the other angle.*

Add the sine of the side given to the sine of the angle opposite to the side required, and from the sum subtract the sine of the angle opposite to the side given, or add its cosecant ; the remainder or sum will be the sine of the side required.

Example. In the triangle szp, having the angle szp 130° 3′ 12″, spz 31° 34′ 26″, and the side zs 40° ; to find the side ps.

9·8080675 sin. zs   40° 0′ 0″
9·8838294 } sin. szp { 49 56 ·
   850 }   { · · 48
0·2808858 } cos. spz { 31 35 ·
   1165 }   { · ·—34
9·9729842 sin. ps reqd. 70 0 0
See pa. 171 following.

Prop. XX. *Having two angles, and a side opposed to one of them ; to find the side between the angles given.*

Let a perpendicular fall from the angle unknown, on its opposite side : then add the cosine of the given angle next the given side, to the tangent of the given side ; the sum (abating radius) is the tangent of the first arc, comprehended between the given angle next the given side, and the segment of the side where the perpendicular falls.

And the second arc, comprehended between the same segment and the other angle, is to be found thus : add the sine of the arc found, to the tangent of the given angle next the given side, and from the sum subtract the tangent of the other angle given, or add its cotangent ; the remainder or sum will be the sine of the second arc.

The sum or difference of these two arcs will be the side required.

Example. In the triangle szp, having the angle zps 31° 34′ 26″, zsp 30° 28′ 12″, and the side pz 38° 30′ ; to find the side sp.

9·9303781 } cos. zps { 31° 35′ ·″
   440 }   { · —34
9·9006052 tan. pz   38 30 0
9·8310273 tan. pr 1st arc 34 7 30
9·7488698 } sin. pr { 34 7
   932 }   { · · 30
9·7884529 } tan. zps { 31 34 ·
   1227 }   { · 26
0·2301404 } cot. zsp { 30 29 ·
   2313 }   { · —48
9·7679103 sin. sr 2d arc 35 52 30
   add pr 1st arc 34 7 30
   sum is sp 70 0 0

See page 171 following.

But when the perpendicular falls out of the triangle, the difference of the two arcs will be the side required.

Prop. XXI. *Having two angles, and a side opposite to one of them ; to find the third angle.*

Let a perpendicular fall from the angle unknown, on its opposite side : then add the cosine of the given side to the tangent of the adjacent angle ; the sum (abating radius) is the cotangent of the first angle to be found, comprehended by the given side and the perpendicular.

And the second angle, comprehended by the perpendicular and the side unknown, is to be found thus : add the sine of the angle found, to the cosine of the given angle opposite to the given side, and from the sum subtract the cos.ne of the other angle given, or add its secant; the remainder or sum will be the sine of the second angle.

The sum or difference of these two angles will be the angle required.

Example. In the triangle szp, having the angle zps 31° 34' 26", zsp 30° 28' 12", and the side pz 38° 30'; to find the angle szp.

9·8935444	cosin. pz	38°	30'	0"
9·7884529 }	tang. zps {	31	34	·
1227 }	{	·	·	26
9·6821200	cot. 1st ∠ pzr	64	18	50

9·9547619 }	sin. pzr {	64	18	·
507 }	{	·	·	50
9·9353948 }	cos. zsp {	30	29	·
594 }	{	·	—48
0·0695413 }	sec. zps {	31	34	·
336 }	{	·	·	26
9·9598447	sin. 2d ∠ szr	65	44	21
	then add 1st ∠ pzr	64	18	50
	the sum is szp	130	3	11

See page 171 following.

But when the perpendicular falls out of the triangle, the difference of the two angles will be the angle required.

Prop. XXII. *Having two sides, and the angle between them; to find either of the other angles.*

Let a perpendicular fall from the unknown angle, which is not required, on its opposite side: then add the cosine of the given angle to the tangent of the given side opposite to the angle required; the sum (abating radius) is the tangent of the first arc, comprehended between the given angle and the segment of the given side where the perpendicular falls.

And the second arc is the difference of that side and the first arc, being comprehended between the same segment and the angle required.

Now add the sine of the first arc, to the tangent of the given angle, and from the sum subtract the sine of the second arc, or add its cosecant; the remainder or sum will be the tangent of the angle required.

Example. In the triangle szp, having the side pz 38° 30', ps 70°, and the angle zps 31° 34' 26"; to find the angle zsp.

9·9303781 }	cosin. zps {	31° 34'	·
440 }	{	·	·	26
9·9006052	tang. pz	38	30	0
9·8310273	tan. pr, 1st arc	34	7	30
	taken from ps	70	0	0
	leaves sr, 2d arc	35	52	30

9·7488698 }	sin. pr {	34	7	·
932 }	{	·	·	30
9·7884529 }	tang. zps {	31	34	·
1227 }	{	·	·	26
0·2320011 }	cosec. sr {	35	53	·
873 }	{	·	—30
9·7696270	tan. zps req.	30	28	12

See page 171 following.

To find both the unknown angles.

Add together the cosecant, or the complement of the sine, of half the sum of the given sides, the sine of half their difference, and the cotangent of half the angle given; the sum (abating radius) is the tangent of half the difference of the angles required.

Add also together the secant, or the complement of the cosine, of half the sum of the given sides, the cosine of half their difference, and the cotangent of half the angle given; the sum (abating radius) is the tangent of half the sum of the angles required.

Then add the half-difference of the angles required, to their half-sum, and you will have the greater angle; and subtract the half-difference from the half-sum, and you will have the lesser angle required, the same as in the former operation.

PS =	70° 0'	Cosec. ½ sum	0·0906719	Sec. ½ sum	0·2334015
PZ =	38 30	Sin. ¼ diff.	9·4336746	Cosin. ¼ diff.	9·9833805
Sum	108 30	Cot. ½ ZPS	10·5486352	Cot. ½ ZPS	10·5486352
Diff.	31 30	T.49°47'30"	10·0729817	T.80°15'42"	10·7654172
¼ Sum	54 15	Half sum of angles required is . .		80° 15' 42"	
¼ Diff.	15 45	Half the difference is		49' 47 30	
∠ ZPS = 31 34 26"		The greater angle SZP is . . .		130 3 12	
½∠ ZPS = 15 47 13		The lesser angle ZSP is, as before,		30 28 12	

Prop. XXIII. *Having two sides, and the angle between them; to find the third side.*

Let a perpendicular fall from either of the angles unknown, on its opposite side: then add the cosine of the given angle, to the tangent of the side from whose end the perpendicular is let fall; the sum (abating radius) is the tangent of the first arc, comprehended between the given angle and the segment of the side where the perpendicular falls.

And the second arc is the difference of that side and the first arc, being comprehended between the same segment and the end of the side required.

Now add the cosine of the second arc, to the cosine of the side from whose end the perpendicular falls, and from the sum subtract the cosine of the first arc found, or add its secant; the remainder or sum will be the cosine of the side required.

Example. In the triangle SZP, having the side PZ 38° 30', PS 70°, and the angle ZPS 31° 34' 26"; to find the side ZS.

9·9303781 }	cosin. ZPS {	31°	35'	."	
440 }	{	.		−34	
9·9006052	tang. PZ .	38	30	0	
9·8310273	tan.PR,1st arc	34	7	30	
	taken from PS	70	0	0	
	leaves SR, 2d arc	35	52	30	
9·9085988 }	cosin. SR {	35	53	.	
457 }	{	.	.	−30	
9·8935444	cosin. PZ	38	30	0	
0·0820236 }	sec. PR {	34	7	.	
428 }	{	.	.	30	
1·8842553	cosin. ZS req.	40	0	0	

See page 171 following.

Prop. XXIV. *Having two sides, and the angle opposite to one of them; to find the angle opposed to the other side.*

Add the sine of the angle given, to the sine of the side opposite to the angle required, and from the sum subtract the sine of the side opposite to the angle given, or add its cosecant; the remainder or sum will be the sine of the angle required.

Example. In the triangle SZP, having the side PS 70°, ZS 40°, and the angle SZP 130° 3' 12"; to find the angle ZPS.

9·8838294 }	sin.sup.SZP {	49°	56'	.″	
850 }	{	.	.	48	
9·8080675	sin. ZS	40	0	0	
0·0270142	cosec. PS	. 70	0	0	
9·7189961	sin. ZPS req.	31	34	26	

See page 171 following.

Prop. XXV. *Having two sides, and the angle opposite to one of them; to find the third side.*

Let a perpendicular fall from the angle between the sides given, on its opposite side: then add the cosine of the angle given, to the tangent of the given side next that angle; the sum (abating radius) is the tangent of the first arc, comprehended between the given angle and the segment of the side where the perpendicular falls.

Now the 2d arc, comprehended between the same segment, and the end of the side required, is to be found thus: add the cosine of the first arc, to the cosine of the given side opposite to the angle given, and from the sum subtract the cosine of the other given side, or add its secant; the remainder or sum will be the cosine of the second arc.

The sum or difference of these two arcs will be the side required.

Example. In the triangle szp, having the side pz 38° 30′, sz 40°, and the angle spz 31° 34′ 26″; to find the side ps.

$$
\left.\begin{array}{l}9 \cdot 9303781 \\ 440\end{array}\right\}\ \text{cos. spz}\ \left\{\begin{array}{lll}31° & 35′ & .″ \\ . & . & -34\end{array}\right.
$$

9·9006052	tan. pz	38	30	0
9·8310273	tang. PR 1st arc	34	·7	30

$$
\left.\begin{array}{l}9 \cdot 9178908 \\ 428\end{array}\right\}\ \text{cosin. PR}\ \left\{\begin{array}{lll}34 & 8 & .″ \\ . & . & -30\end{array}\right.
$$

9·8842540	cosin. sz .	40	0	0
0·1064556	sec. pz .	38	30	0
9·9086432	cosin. sr 2d arc	35	52	30
	add PR, 1st arc	34	7	30
	gives ps req.	70	0	0

See page 171 following.

But when the perpendicular falls out of the triangle, the difference of the two arcs will be the side required.

Prop. XXVI. *Having two sides, and the angle opposed to one of them; to find the angle between them.*

Let a perpendicular fall from the angle between the sides given, on its opposite side: then add the cosine of the given side next the given angle, to the tangent of that angle; the sum (abating radius) is the cotangent of the first angle to be found, comprehended by the given side next the angle given, and by the perpendicular.

Now the second angle, comprehended by the perpendicular and the other given side, is to be found thus: add the cosine of the first angle found, to the tangent of the given side next the angle given, and from the sum subtract the tangent of the other given side, or add its cotangent; the remainder or sum will be the cosine of the second angle to be found.

The sum or the difference of the first and second angles, will be the angle required.

Example. In the triangle szp, having the side pz 38° 30′, sz 40°, and the angle spz 31° 34′ 26″; to find the angle szp.

9·8935444	cosin. pz	38°	30′	0″

$$
\left.\begin{array}{l}9 \cdot 7884529 \\ 1227\end{array}\right\}\ \text{tang. szp}\ \left\{\begin{array}{lll}31 & 34 & . \\ . & . & 26\end{array}\right.
$$

9·6821200	cotan. pzr, 1st ∠	64	18	50

$$
\left.\begin{array}{l}9 \cdot 6368859 \\ 437\end{array}\right\}\ \text{cosin. pzr}\ \left\{\begin{array}{lll}64 & ·19 & .″ \\ . & . & -10\end{array}\right.
$$

9·9006052	tang. pz .	38	30	0
0·0761865	cotan. sz .	40	0	0
9·6137213	cosin. szr, 2d ∠	65	44	22
	add pzr, 1st ∠	64	18	50
	gives szp, req.	130	3	12

See page 171 following.

Prop. XXVII. *Having two angles, and the side between them; to find either of the other sides.*

Let a perpendicular fall from the given angle, which is next the side required, upon its opposite side: then add the cosine of the given side to the tangent of the given angle opposite to the side required; the sum (abating radius) is the cotangent of the first angle to be found, comprehended by the given side and the perpendicular.

And the second angle is the difference between the first and the given angle next the required side, being comprehended by the perpendicular and that side.

Now add the cosine of the first angle found, to the tangent of the side given, and from the sum subtract the cosine of the second angle, or add its secant; the remainder or sum will be the tangent of the side required.

Example. In the triangle szp, having the angle spz 31° 34′ 26″, szp 130° 3′ 12″, and the side pz 38° 30′; to find the side sz.

9·8935444 cosin. PZ - 38° 30′ 0″
9·7884529 } tang. SPZ { 31 34 .
    1227 }   { . . 26
9·6821200 cot. PZR, 1st ∠, 64 18 50
    taken from SZP 130 3 12
    leaves SZR, 2d ∠, 65 44 22
9·6368859 } cosin. PZR { 64 19 .
     437 }   { . .—10
9·9006052 tang. PZ - 38 30 0
0·3861750 } sec. SZR. { 65 44 .
    1028 }   { . . 22
9·9238126 tan. sz req. 40 0 0

See page 171 following.

To find both the unknown sides.

Add together the cosecant, or the complement of the sine, of half the sum of the angles given, the sine of half their difference, and the tangent of half the given side; the sum (abating radius) is the tangent of half the difference of the sides required.

Add also together the secant, or the complement of the cosine, of half the sum of the given angles, the cosine of half their difference, and the tangent of half the given side; the sum (abating radius) is the tangent of half the sum of the sides required.

Then add half the difference of the sides required, to their half-sum, and you will have the greater side; and subtract the half-difference from the half-sum, and you will have the lesser side required, the same as in the former operation.

SZP	130° 3′ 12″	Cosec. ½ sum 0·0056062	Sec. ½ sum 0·7968360
SPZ	31 34 26	Sin. ½ diff. 9·8793527	Cosin. ½ diff. 9·8148437
Sum	161 37 38	Tang. ½ PZ 9 5430936	Tang. ½ PZ 9·5430936
Diff.	98 28 46	Tang. of 15° 9·4280525	Tang. of 55° 10·1547733
½ Sum	80 48 49	Half sum of the sides required is - - - 55°	
½ Diff.	49 14 23	Half their difference is - - - - - 15	
PZ	38 30 0	The greater side SP is - - - - - 70	
½ PZ	19 15 0	Lesser side sz is, as before - - - - 40	

Prop. XXVIII. *Having two angles and the side between them; to find the third angle.*

Let a perpendicular fall from either of the angles given, upon its opposite side: then add the cosine of the side given to the tangent of the given angle, from which the perpendicular does not fall; the sum (abating radius) is the cotangent of the first angle, comprehended by the given side and the perpendicular.

And the second angle is the difference between the first and the given angle that the perpendicular fell from, being comprehended by the perpendicular and the side opposite to the other angle given.

Now add the sine of the second angle to the cosine of that given angle from which the perpendicular did not fall, and from the sum subtract the sine of the first angle found, or add its cosecant; the remainder or sum will be the cosine of the angle required.

Example. In the triangle SZP, having the angle SZP 130° 3′ 12″, SPZ 31° 34′ 26″, and the side PZ 38° 30′; to find the angle PSZ.

9·8935444 cosin. PZ - 38 30 0
9·7884529 } tang. SPZ { 31 34 .
    1227 }   { . . 26
9·6821200 cotan. PZR, 1st ∠, 64 18 50
    taken from SZP 130 3 12
    leaves SZR, 2d ∠, 65 44 22
0·0451773 } cosec. PZR { 64 19 .
     101 }   { . . —10
9·9303781 } cosin. SPZ { 31 35 .
     440 }   { . . —34
9·9598246 } sin. SZR { 65 44 .
     209 }   { . . 22
9·9354550 cosin. PSZ req. 30 28 0

See page 171 following.

Z

FOR THE USE OF THE VERSED SINES MAY BE ALSO ADDED THE FOLLOWING PROPOSITIONS.

Prop. I. Having two sides of a spheric triangle, with the angle between them; to find the third side.

ADD together the log. versed sine of the contained angle, and the log. sines of the two sides; the sum (abating twice the radius) is the logarithm of a number to be found, which added to the natural versed sine of the difference of the two given sides, the sum will be the natural versed sine of the third side sought.

Or when the contained angle is above 90°, add the log. versed sine of its supplement, and the log. sines of the two sides together; the sum (abating twice the radius) is the logarithm of a number to be found, and subtracted from the natural versed sine of the sum of the two given sides, the remainder will be the natural versed sine of the third side sought.

Example 1. In the triangle s z P, having the side PZ 38° 30′, PS 70°, and the angle ZPS 31° 34′ 26″; to find the side zs.
9·1703625 log.ver.sine zPP 31° 34′ 26″
9·7941496 log. sine of PZ 38 30 0
9·9729858 log. sine of PS 70 0 0
8·9374979 log. of the numb. 865960
Nat. vers. diff. sides 31° 30′ 1473598
Nat. vers. zs 40° - - - 2339558

Example 2. In the triangle s z P, having the side PZ 38° 30′, zs 40°, and the angle szP 130° 3′ 12″; to find the side PS.

The angle vzP is the supplement of szP.

9·5520590 log. vers. vzP 49° 56′ 48″
9·7941496 log. sin. PZ 38 30 0
9·8080675 log. sin. zs 40 0 0
9·1542761 log.of the number 1426514
Nat. vers. sum sides 78° 30′ 8006321
Nat. vers. PS 70° - - - 6579807

This proposition may be very useful in finding the distances of places on the earth, whose longitudes and latitudes are known; the distances of stars, whose declinations and right ascensions, or longitudes and latitudes, are known; and consequently the altitudes, or common altitude of two stars, or two altitudes of the sun, and time between the observations, or difference of azimuth, being taken, the latitude of the place may readily be found.

Prop. II. Having two angles of a spheric triangle, and the side between them; to find the third angle.

Let the angles be changed into sides, and the side into an angle; then proceed as in the former proposition, and the result will be the supplement of the third angle. But if one of the given angles exceed 90°, take its supplement, and the result will be the third angle.

The following remarks and directions, for rendering the proportional part of a logarithm always additive, and for using $c + t$, $c—t$, &c, for s or c &c, in the foregoing propositions, 20, 21, 22, 23, 25, 26, 27, 28, were communicated by the Rev. Nevil Maskelyne, D. D. astronomer royal, and F. R. S. the fourth case having been invented by him many years since, and delivered to the computors of the Nautical Ephemeris, as precepts necessary in computing the moon's distance from the stars in some cases, and the rest he has now added on this occasion.

" The result of trigonometrical calculations will be sometimes inaccurate, owing to the logarithms not being carried to a greater number of places in the table, as will sufficiently appear from the logarithmic differences being small. This will happen where the answer comes out in the cosine of a very small angle, or the sine of an angle near 90°. The greatness of the differences of the log. sines of small arcs, or cosines of large ones, will sometimes affect the accuracy of the result of the second part of the operation, unless the first arc be found to a small part of a minute or second: To prevent such error, and render the computation easier, putting t, t', s, c for the tangent, cotangent, sine, and cosine of the 1st arc or angle, then in the 2d part of the work,

In Prop. 20, if the first arc	is very small,	for s use $c + t$
21 - - - angle	is very small,	for s use $c — t'$
22 - - - arc	is very small,	for s use $c + t$
23 - - - arc	is near 90°,	for—c use $t — s$
25 - - - arc	is near 90°,	for c use $s — t$
26 - - - angle	is near 90°,	for c use $s + t'$
27 - - - angle	is near 90°,	for c use $s + t'$
28 - - - angle	is very small,	for—s use $t' — c$

This obviates the necessity of finding the first arc to a very minute exactness, which otherwise would be necessary in taking out the sine or cosine of the same arc in the second part of the work.

Where the foregoing precepts direct to subtract a sine or cosine, it will be readier in practice to add a cosecant or secant; and where they direct to subtract a tangent (which is done in prop. 26) it will be readier to add a cotangent. This method being used, if it be required to find the logarithmic sines, &c, to the exactness of a second, and the logarithm is increasing (as in the sines, tangents, and secants), write down the logarithm for the degree and minute without the seconds; and also write down the proportional part for the seconds; but, if the logarithm is decreasing (as in the cosines, cotangents, and cosecants) write down the logarithm for the next greater minute, and also write down the proportional part for the complement of the seconds to 60; and proceed in like manner

Z 2

with every logarithmic sine, cosine, &c, used in the work; the sum of all the logarithms (abating one or two radii or tens in the index, according as 2 or 3 logarithmic sines, &c are used in the part of the work in question) will be the logarithmic sine, cosine, tangent, or cotangent required.

Ex. 1. To find the log. sine of 34° 17′ 24″
Here log. sine of 34° 17′ - - 9·7507287
And as 60 : 24 or as 10 : 4 : : 1853 : - 741
         9·7508028

Ex. 2. To find the log. cos. of 55° 42′ 36″
Log. cos. of 55° 43′ - - - 9·7507287
60 : 24 (60—36), or 10 : 4 : : 1853 : - 741
         9·7508028

Ex. 3. In the triangle PLS, given

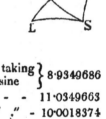

P = 20° 30′ 48″
PS = 85 3 40 to find LS by prop. 23;
PL = 89 10 0 SD being perp. PL.

P 20° 31′ .″ cos. - 9·9715404
 . —12 - - - - - 95
PS 85 3 . tan. 11·0624350 } cos. found by taking } 8·9349686
 . . 40 - - - - - 9814 } tang. from sine }
PD 84 43 43 tan. 11·0349663 - - · - - - 11·0349663
PL 89 10 0   cosec. PD 84° 44′ .″ - 10·0018374
LD 4 26 17   — 17 -   33
        cosin. LD 4 27 . - 9·9986888
          — 43 -   70
       cosin. LS 20 53 24 - 9·9704714

Here to avoid the trouble of finding the proportional part for the large logarithm difference of the cosine of PS, that cosine is found by subtracting the tangent of it (already found) from the sine, which is easily found, because the differences are small: And, for the same reason, the sum of the tangent and cosecant of PD, are used instead of its secant.

N. B. The perpendicular should always be let fall from the end of the side, PS or PL, which differs most from 90°, over or under."

OF THE TRAVERSE TABLE.

THIS traverse table, or table of difference of latitude and departure, in page 338 and 339, is so contrived, as to have the whole in one view; and is so plainly titled as to want little or no explanation.

The distances 1, 2, 3, &c, at the top and bottom, may be accounted 10, 20, 30, &c, and the 10 as 100, if the minutes of latitude and departure answering to the course be increased in the same proportion; so that if the distance consists of two significant figures, the difference of latitude, and the departure, is each to be taken out at twice; and if of three figures, at thrice.

The chief design of this table, is for the ready and exact working of traverses; but it may also be applied to the solution of the several cases of plain sailing, and to some other uses.

Prop. I. *Having the course and distance, to find the difference of latitude and departure.*

Seek the course on the left hand of both pages downwards, if less than four points, or 45 degrees; or if greater, on the right hand upwards; and even with it in the double column, signed at the top and bottom with the distance, is found both the difference of latitude and the departure.

Example 1. A ship sails ssw ¾ w 37 miles; the difference of latitude and the departure are required.

Find the course 2¼ points on the left-hand side of each page, and even with it in the double columns signed 3, and 7, the two figures of the distance, the difference of latitude for 30 is 25·732, and for 7 is 6·004, the sum is 31·736 for the whole difference of latitude; and the departure for 30 is 15·423, and for 7 is 3·599, the sum is 19·022 for the whole departure.

Thus, Dist.		Diff. Lat.	Dep.
30	- -	25·732 -	15·423
7	- -	6·004 -	3·599
37 miles		31·736 -	19·022

Example 2. A ship sails se 49° 148 miles; the difference of latitude and the departure are required.

Find the course 49 degrees on the right-hand side of each page, and even with it in the double columns signed 10, 4, and 8, the difference of latitude at 100 miles is 65·606, at 40 is 26.242. and at 8 is 5·248; the sum is 97·096 for the whole difference of latitude. And the departure at 100 miles is 75·471, at 40 is 30·188, and

at 8 is 6·038; the sum is 111·697 for the whole departure. Thus,

Dist.	Diff. Lat.	Depart.
100 - - -	65.606 -	75·471
40 - - -	26·242 -	30·188
8 - - -	5·248 -	6·038
148 miles	97·096 -	111·697

Prop. II. *Having several courses and distances; to find the difference of latitude and the departure.*

Make a table in the following manner, and put therein each course and distance; then find the difference of latitude and departure to each course by the preceding, and place them in the proper column; the difference of the sums of the northings and southings, is the whole difference of latitude; and the difference of the sums of the eastings and westings, is the whole departure.

Example. A ship from the latitude of 50° north, sails according to the courses and distances set in the traverse table; the differences of latitude, and the departure, are found at the bottom.

THE TRAVERSE TABLE.

Courses.	Dist. Miles.	Diff. of Lat. North.	South.	Departure. East.	West.
S S E ½ E	79		69·671	37·241	
S E ½ E	86		54·557	66·479	
S b W ½ W	109		101·687		36·384
S 48° W	112		74·942		83·231
N 58° W	70	6·101			59·734
S 40° W	84		64·348		53·994
		6·101	365·205	103·720	243·343
			6·101		103·720
Diff. la. 359·104			359·104	Depart. 139·623	139·623

This proposition may be applied in the surveying of large tracts of land, as a county, &c. and was made use of by Mr. Norwood in measuring the distance from York to London, as the road led him, observing the several bearings by his circumferentor, and finding by such a table his several differences of latitude, and departure, by which he obtained the distance between the parallels of London and York, pretty near the truth, so long ago as the year 1635; as may be seen in his Seaman's Practice.

Also in plotting the survey of a county thus taken, the circuit station-lines, though consisting of many hundreds, may be reduced to a few for the first closing, and the like for the intermediates of each line first plotted, by which every station may perhaps be more truly placed than by any other method: the distances in the table may be chains of 66, or 100 feet, as well as miles, or any other measure that the differences of latitude and departure would be had in.

Prop. III. *Having the difference of latitude, and the departure; to find the course and distance.*

Seek the given difference of latitude and departure, taken together, in their columns, or the nearest numbers to them; and the course is even therewith at the side, and the distance at the top and bottom: but if the given difference of latitude and departure cannot be found nearly, take $\frac{1}{2}$, $\frac{1}{3}$, &c. part, or any equal multiple of them that can be found; then the course is even with them at the side, and such a part of the distance, as was taken of the difference of latitude and departure, at the top and bottom.

Example 1. Given the difference of latitude 59 miles s, and the departure 68 miles w; the course and distance are required.

In the double column over 9, even with 49° at the right-hand side, is

found together the given difference of latitude and departure; therefore the course is 49° sw, and the distance 90 miles.

Example 2. Given the difference of latitude 30 miles N, and the departure 18 miles E; the course and distance are required.

Here the given difference of latitude and departure, or any numbers near them, are not to be found together in the table; therefore taking $\frac{1}{2}$ or the double of each, the course is found to be 31° N E, and the distance 35 miles.

Note. A table computed to every mile in the distance up to 100 miles would more readily solve this example.

Prop. IV. *Having the departure and middle latitude; to find the difference of longitude, according to the method used by* W. Jones, Esq. F. R. S.

Seek the given departure, or the next less number in the columns signed lat. even with the middle given latitude found among the courses, and at the top and bottom (signed dist.) is the difference of longitude sought; which, if not found directly at once, may be taken out at twice or thrice.

Example 1. Being yesterday noon in the latitude of 37° 17′ N, and this day noon in 38° 43′ N, and by the table the departure is found 70·921 E; the difference of longitude is required.

In the column signed lat. under 9, even with 38°, the middle latitude is found 7·0921; therefore 90 miles is the difference of longitude sought.

Example 2. Being yesterday noon in latitude 46° 25′ N, and this day at noon in 47° 35′ N, so that the middle latitude is 47° N, and the departure is found 112·53 miles w; required the difference of longitude.

In the column signed lat. over 10 at the bottom, even with 47 at the right-hand side, is 6·8200; therefore subducting 68·200 from 112·53, the remainder is 44·33; then over 6 is 4·0920, and 40·92 subducted from 44·33 leaves 3·41, which is found over 5; therefore the difference of longitude is 165 miles west.

If the middle latitude be not an even degree, but have odd minutes; find the difference of longitude, for the even degrees next less and greater, and add a proportional part of the difference between the two results to the lesser; the sum will be the difference of longitude sought.

Suppose the middle latitude in the last example had been 47° 20′ N, then, after finding the difference of longitude as before for 47°, find it also for 48°, which is 168 miles; then ⅓ of the difference being added to the former, gives the difference of longitude 166 miles west.

Note. Though this method is not in all cases near the truth, yet when the miles are geographical, it is sufficiently near for daily practice in any voyage, as well as easy, and very expeditious.

Prop. V. *Having the latitudes and the longitudes of two places, to find the bearing and distance.*

Seek the complement of the middle latitude among the degrees, and the difference of longitude in minutes among the distances, the departure answering is found in its proper column; then with the difference of latitude and departure, find their bearing or course and distance by the third.

Example. Let the Lizard be given in the latitude of 49, 50′ N, and 5° 21′ w longitude, and Cape Ortegal in the latitude of 44° 10′ N, and 7¼° 43′ w longitude; to find the bearing and distance.

The difference of longitude is 142′; and in the columns signed dep. under 10, 4, and 2, even with 43° the co-middle latitude, are found 6·8200, 2·7280, and 1·3640; then increasing the two former as before shown, their sum is 96·844 miles w, for the departure; and the bearing, or course, answering to 340 miles difference of latitude, with 96·844 departure, is found about 16° sw: and the distance about 354 miles.

OF MERCATOR'S SAILING.

THE uses of the table of meridional parts are fully supplied by the table of logarithmic tangents, as is demonstrated in N° 219 of the Philosophical Transactions. It is there proved, 1st, That the meridional line, or scale of Mercator's Chart, is a scale of the log. tangents of the half-complements of the latitude. 2dly, That such log. tangents of Mr. Briggs's form, are a scale of the differences of longitude, on the rumb which makes an angle of 51° 38′ 9″ with the meridian. And 3dly, That the differences of longitude on different rumbs, are to one another as the tangents of the angles of those rumbs with the meridian.

Hence it follows, that the difference of the log. tangents of the half complements of the latitudes, is to the difference of longitude a ship makes in sailing on any rumb from the one latitude to the other, as the tangent of 51° 38′ 9″ (whose logarithm is 10·1015104) to the tangent of the angle of the rumb or course with the meridian; so that:

I. If two latitudes, and the difference of longitude, be given, the course and distance are readily determined by this rule.

Take, by help of the tables, the difference of the log. tangents of the half-complements of the latitudes, esteeming the last three figures to be a decimal fraction; and add the complement of its logarithm to the logarithm of the difference of longitude reduced to minutes, and the constant log. 10·1015104; the sum (abating radius) shall be the log. tangent of the course. And to the log. secant of the course, add the logarithm of the difference of latitude reduced to minutes, the sum (abating radius) shall be the logarithm of the distance in minutes.

Example. Given the Lizard to be in latitude 49° 55′ N, Barbadoes in 13° 10′ N, and their difference of longitude 53° 00′, or 3180′ W; to find the course and distance.

½ Co. lat. $\begin{cases} \text{Barbadoes } 38^\circ\ 25'\ \text{l. tan. } 9\cdot8993082\ \text{l. } 3180' = 3\cdot5024271 \\ \text{Lizard } \quad 20 \quad\ 2\frac{1}{2}\ \text{l. tan. } 9\cdot5620477\ \text{const. log. } 10\cdot1015104 \end{cases}$

diff. 3372·605 its co. log. 6·4720346

Log. tang. of the course 49° 59′ 10″ sw - - - - - - 10·0759721

Log. sec. of the course 49 59 10 - - - - - - - 10·1918067

Log. of 2205′ diff. of the latitudes - - - - - - - 3·3434086

Log. of 3429·378 distance of Barbadoes from the Lizard   3·5352153

II. If two latitudes and the course be given, the difference of longitude is obtained with the same ease: for as the tangent of 51° 38′ 9″ is to the tangent of the course, so is the difference of the log. tangents of the half-complements of the latitudes, to the difference of longitude sought. Therefore, to the complement of the constant log. 10·1015104, add the log. of the difference of the log. tangents of the half-complements of the latitudes, and the log. tangent of the course, the sum (abating radius) will be the log. of the difference of longitude in minutes.

Example. Given the latitudes 49° 55′ and 13° 10′, and course 49° 59′ 10″; to find the difference of longitude.

Lat. 13° 10′, its ½co.lat. 38° 25′ l. tan. 9·8993082

Lat. 49 55 - - - 20 2½ l.tan. 9·5620477 co.const.log. 9·8984896

diff. 3372·605 - its log. 3·5279654

Log. tang. of the course 49° 59′ 10″ - - - - - - 10·0759721

Log. of 3180′ = 53° for diff. of longitude - - - - 3·5024271

By this rule, having two good observations of the latitude, and the course duly steered, the reckoning of a ship's way is best ascertained, especially if you sail near the meridian.

III. If the latitude departed from, the course steered, and distance sailed, be given; to find the ship's latitude, and difference of longitude.

First, the latitude is obtained from the consideration that the distance is to the difference of latitude, as radius to the cosine of the course, which is common to plain sailing. Therefore to the log. of the distance add the log. cosine of the course, the sum (abating radius) is the log. of the difference of latitudes; which difference added to the lesser latitude, or subtracted from the greater, the sum or remainder is the present latitude: then having the two latitudes and the course, the difference of longitude is found by the second.

Example. Having sailed from the Lizard, in lat. 49₀ 55′ N, on a course 49° 59′ 10″ south-westerly 3429·378 miles : required what longitude and latitude the ship is found in.

Log. of 3429·378 the distance sailed .... 3·5352153
Log. cosine of 49° 59′ 10″ the course .... 9·8081933
Log. of 2205′, or 36° 45′ diff. of the latitudes .... 3·3434086

Now subtracting 36° 45′ from 49° 55′, the remainder 13° 10′ N, is the latitude the ship is found in.

By which latitude, now known, the difference of log. tangents will be found 3372·605, and the further process in nothing differing from the second rule, by which the difference of longitude will be found 53° 00′.

Thus the dead reckoning by the log line, and daily account of a ship's way, are duly kept, and the trouble very little more than by plain sailing.

These are all the cases that occur in practice; the rest, which are mostly speculative, are either easily reducible to these, or else not to be performed by logarithms, and therefore come not at present under our cognizance.

But it is to be noted, that both the complements of the latitudes are to be estimated from the same pole of the world; which may be from either; and therefore if one latitude be N, and the other S, to have their complements, you must add 90° to one of them, and subtract the other from 90, and then the operation will be the same as in the preceding cases.

Example. Given St. Jago, one of the Cape-de-Verd islands, in the latitude of 14° 56′ N; and the island St. Helena, in latitude 15° 45′ S, and their difference of longitude 30° 12′ E; to find the course and distance.

ℓ Co. lat. { St. Jago   52° 28′. l. tan. 10·1144965   l. 1812′ 3·2581582
{ St. Helena 37. 7¼.   l. tan. 9·8790845 const. log. 10·1015104

                2354·120 its co. log. 6·6281714

Log. tang. of the course 44° 11′ 53″ SE .... 9·9878400
Log. sec. of the course 44 11 53 .... 10·1445200
Log. of 1841′ diff. of the latitudes .... 3·2650538
Log. of 2567·875 distance of St. Helena from St. Jago .... 3·4095738

Or if it be thought easier, when one latitude is N, and the other S, you may add 90° to each of them, the sum of the log. tangents of their halves (abating twice the radius) will be the same as the difference of the log. tangents of the former. For an example, take the same latitudes as in the preceding.

Then 90° + { 14° 56′ = 104° 56′ } its half { 52° 28′ l. tan. 10·1144965
           { 15 45 = 105 45 }   { 52 52¼ l. tan. 10·1209155

The sum (abating twice the radius) equal to the former distance .... 2354·120

Also, when both latitudes are of the same name, that is both N or both S, you may add 90° to each of them, the difference of the log. tangents of half these sums will be the same as of the log. tangents of half the complements of those latitudes.

TABLE FOR THE LENGTHS OF CIRCULAR ARCS.

THIS is table 12, and constitutes page 340. It contains the lengths of every single degree up to 180, and of every minute, second, and third, each up to 60. The form of it is obvious ; the length of each degree, minute, second or third, immediately following it on the same line in the next column. And the two following examples will show the use of the table.

Ex. 1. To find the length of an arc of 57° 17′ 44″ 48‴.

Take out from their respective columns the lengths answering to each of these numbers singly, and add them all together, thus :

57° . . .	0·9948377
17′ . . .	49451
44″ . . .	2133
48‴ . . .	39

the sum or   1·0000000   is the whole length, and is equal to the radius; that is, the length of an arc of 57° 17′ 44″ 48‴ is equal to the radius of the circle.

Ex. 2. To find the degrees, minutes, &c in the arc 1, which is equal to the radius.

Subtract from it the next less tabular arc, and from the remainder the next less again, and so on till nothing remain; and opposite to the several numbers subtracted, will be the degree, minutes, &c ; thus :

Given length	1·0000000
57°	0.9948377
	51623
17′	49451
	2172
44″ . . .	2133
48‴	39

So that the arc which is equal to the radius contains 57° 17′ 44″ 48‴.

TABLE FOR COMPARING HYP. AND COMMON LOGS.

THIS is table 13, and is the upper part of page 341. It contains the hyperbolic logs. answering to the first 100 common logs. and is very useful for speedily changing the one into the other.

Ex. 1. To find the hyp. log. answering to the common log. 0·9542425.

Beginning at the left hand, and dividing the given number into periods of two figures each, including the index, take out the hyp. log. to each period, omitting two figures at the 2d period, four at the third, and six at the 4th; then add them all together, thus:

com. log.		hyp. log.
09	. .	2·0723266
54	. .	1243396
24	. .	5526
25	.	58
0·9542425		2·1972246 ans.

Ex. 2. To find the common log. answering to the hyp. log. 2.1972246.

Subtract continually each next less tabular hyp. log. from the given number, and from the remainders; and the several common logarithms answering to these tabular hyp. logs, joined together, will be the com. log. required, thus:

		hyp. log.
given		2·1972246
09	. . .	2·0723226
		1248980
54	. . .	1243396
		5584
24	. . .	5526
		58
25	. .	58
0·9542425 answer.		

The remaining pages contain the small table of the names and degrees, &c, in the points of the compass; which needs no illustration; and a copious list of such errors, with their corrections, as have been discovered in the principal books of logarithms; among which are many that have been detected by myself, both in the Avignon edition of Gardiner, and in Gardiner's own quarto edition, as well as in the French tables by Callet, and by Didot; which renders this list more complete than any former one; and it will be found very useful in correcting those books of tables which are already in the possession of the public. As to all the editions of Sherwin's and Gardiner's tables in octavo, the errors in them are far too numerous to be printed in this or any other work, as they amount to many thousands, even in the edition of 1742, published by Gardiner, in which the last figures of the logarithms are usually not correct to the nearest unit, except in a very few pages at the beginning, and at the end of the table, so that it cannot be depended on for nice calculations.

THE NEW YORK PUBLIC LIBRARY
REFERENCE DEPARTMENT

This book is under no circumstances to be
taken from the Building

form 410

CPSIA information can be obtained
at www.ICGtesting.com
Printed in the USA
BVHW060426100621
609091BV00011B/1117